Praise for *Fit Soul, Fit Body*

"There's no question Mark and Brant know how to get people into the best shape of their lives—both mentally and physically. They've been motivating and inspiring people for decades. And with this book they bring all their knowledge and insights together in a brilliant, one-of-a-kind volume. Read it, apply it, and it will change your life!"

—Michael Besancon, Senior Global Vice President, Whole Foods Market

"Mark Allen and Brant Secunda unite the worlds of physical achievement and spiritual peace in this timely guide that should have its own section in the bookstore called 'Can't Live Without It!'"

—Al Trautwig, NBC Sports Broadcaster and Olympic Commentator

"World-class athlete Mark Allen and shaman healer Brant Secunda join forces to create a unique, practical, and inspired approach to lasting fitness. Combining physical/emotional awareness with ancient spiritual practices is brilliant! *Fit Soul, Fit Body* is a fascinating read."

—Lilias Folan, Master Yoga Teacher, PBS Host

"I have appreciated Brant Secunda's extraordinary wisdom over the years and we are blessed that he and Mark Allen have combined their knowledge into this very special book. The focus on training our bodies has long been hungry for this integration of Spirit into the topic. Thank you, Brant and Mark, for integrating these special concepts that you are so competent to do, these concepts that have application to health, illness, and well-being."

—O. Carl Simonton, MD, Author of Bestsellers *Getting Well Again* and *The Healing Journey*, Medical Director of the Simonton Cancer Center

"Brant and Mark present an exceptional and creative combination of physical and spiritual practices. Ancient and timeless wisdom unites health research and programs for real change. Personal stories and helpful instructions by both authors will lead any reader into the center of his or her basic questions and to long-lasting effective solutions. Absolutely authentic, outstanding, and incomparable!"

—Prof. Dr. Gerhard Marcel Martin, Author of Fourteen Books, Including *Fest: A Celebration of Life*, Marburg University, Germany and Otani University, Kyoto, Japan

FIT SOUL   FIT BODY

FIT SOUL ❧ FIT BODY

— 9 Keys to a Healthier, Happier You —

Brant Secunda and Mark Allen

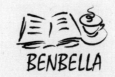

BENBELLA BOOKS, INC.
Dallas, TX

Copyright © 2008 by Brant Secunda and Mark Allen

BenBella Books, Inc.
6440 N. Central Expressway, Suite 503
Dallas, TX 75206
www.benbellabooks.com
Send feedback to feedback@benbellabooks.com

Printed in the United States of America
10 9 8 7 6 5 4 3 2 1

Library of Congress Cataloging-in-Publication Data is available for this title.
ISBN 978-1933771-56-4

Proofreading by Stacia Seaman
Cover design by Laura Watkins
Text design and composition by PerfecType, Nashville, TN
Printed by Bang Printing

Cover Photos:
Waterfall © Diane Cook and Len Jenshel/Getty Images
Woman © Tim Robberts/Getty Images
Man © Steve Bonini/Getty Images
Children © Ryan McVay/Getty Images

For special sales contact Robyn White at robyn@benbellabooks.com

Acknowledgments

We would like to acknowledge BenBella and Glenn Yeffeth for their support of *Fit Soul, Fit Body*. We want to extend a special thanks to Kristin Loberg for her insight and skill that helped make this book what it is.

Dedication

To my Huichol grandfather, Don José Matsuwa.
I give thanks for his trust, love, and our close companionship.
I also dedicate this book to the Great Spirit of Creation.

Brant Secunda

To my teacher and coauthor, Brant Secunda.
It is because of his immense help and guidance, powerful blessings,
incredibly positive energy, and profound wisdom that
I have these stories to share with you.

Mark Allen

Foreword

By Stephen R. Covey

"No work equals no results." I couldn't agree more with that statement, which Mark Allen shared in a thrilling talk he gave at an event for FranklinCovey a few years back. We were in Hawaii to celebrate our top producers for the company, and I found myself clinging enthusiastically onto every word that came out of Mark's mouth . . . waiting for more of his story and a chance to dig deeper into his treasure chest. His clear edge came through the help of his teacher, Brant Secunda, who introduced Mark to the idea of having both a Fit Body and a Fit Soul. I was so moved by his presentation that I walked straight up to him afterward to introduce myself. Clearly, anyone who can win the Ironman World Championship, much less six in a row, has got to have some secrets. I was surprised by how incredibly universal Mark's message was, because the only Ironman I am interested in mastering is that of life—of self- and community leadership. Well, let me tell you, what you hold in your hands is a guide to that kind of Ironman.

Mark Allen had more than the usual run-of-the-mill tale of triumph. This was a man who was unstoppable *not* because he was physically the best, but because he was emotionally and spiritually at the top of his game. Aside from the typical sacrifices made and the adversities overcome, he had learned, under the tutelage of the renowned shaman Brant Secunda, *how to train his mind alongside his body*. I knew that the two would team up and write a book someday to reveal their nuggets of wisdom. What Mark gained from Brant's guidance led to his profound metamorphosis, not only as a world-class athlete, but also—and more important—as a human being.

Brant's stories of transformation and personal change are equally gripping and engaging, from his incredible tale of trekking from New Jersey to the Sierra Madre Mountains of Mexico, where he lived with the Huichol natives for more than a decade, to his sage advice on tapping unlikely sources of strength based on Huichol tradition. These two men are a force to be reckoned with in the world of transformational leadership. They are the consummate teachers about how to develop yourself physically and mentally to live your best life. To instigate and adapt to change. To evolve holistically using a principle-centered approach, which echoes how I've always coached people to reach their peak potential. This book is guaranteed to motivate and inspire you in ways you never thought possible, just as I experienced that day in Hawaii.

Personal transformation is exactly what this book is about. By "personal transformation," I am referring to becoming a better, fitter person in every sense of that word *fit*. And as you'll soon learn, being "fit" has less to do with your heart rate than it has to do with becoming a more effective individual overall—at work, at home, when faced with challenges, and when trying to get more done or take your life to the next level. In fact, when you look up the word fit in the dictionary, you'll find that the first definition states, "adapted to a purpose." Mark and Brant return us to that fundamental meaning, which has been long forgotten on so many levels in modern society.

This book could very well be its own habit in my bestselling book, *The 7 Habits of Highly Effective People*. I'd call it "Embrace the Wisdom of Mark Allen and Brant Secunda." Seriously. Their philosophy is perfectly aligned with most of what I've ever taught. They are a living example of what it means to be fit from the inside out, from the depths of the inner spirit to the outer symbols of health and wellness. All of which then feed accomplishment, self-confidence, and success. At the core of their message is the concept of preserving and nourishing a vibrant and enriched soul—the soul that we all possess no matter our personal credo or religious practices. The physical body, after all, is merely a reflection of all that goes on at a microscopic and often metaphysical level. A fit body is predicated on a fit soul—the emotional part of you that responds to experiences and serves as the trusty glue between your body and mind.

Among the questions Mark and Brant address that I think you will find as illuminating as I have are: Where will we draw strength from when we want to quit? Are we the person our dreams demand us to be to achieve them? You will be amazed by the nuggets of wisdom Mark and Brant reveal in their book, and which can help you to do or change anything you want in life. Don't for a moment think this is only about your health. It's about everything that makes *you*— your passion and enthusiasm for life. Your ability to achieve. Your ambitions, hopes, dreams, and goals. Your relationships, both with others as well as with yourself. Your capacity to stave off stress and optimize your environment so you can usher in physical, spiritual, and emotional well-being. And, of course, your wherewithal to participate in life to its fullest and be happy.

We live in a world where we can no longer separate "business" from the pleasure of personal health. It's true, as Mark and Brant teach, *You can only do so much with the body and so much more with the mind.* Examples of people who are in tip-top physical shape but who fail in their personal and professional lives abound, and the same holds true of people who "have it all" in their personal and professional lives yet who struggle physically. I regularly encounter people who seemingly do everything right—they work hard, they educate themselves and continue to learn new things to propel their career, they have loving families and friendships and live in a supportive community to which they contribute, they seek new opportunities and grab at good ones, they have no addictions or "bad" habits, they strive to take care of their bodies and pay attention to diet and exercise, and on and on . . . but at the end of the day they still feel dissatisfied, off-kilter to some degree, and not living their absolute best. If you were to ask them how "well" they really are, they'd hesitate. And if you were to ask them to put a number on the quality of their lives from 1 to 10 (10 being the best), they'd come in somewhere around 7, maybe 8. What would it be like to live at a throttling 10?

Have you ever had that nagging feeling that something is missing from your life that would bring balance and a sense of completeness? It would put you in control of your life and your potential to realize your greatness. Well, my friends, I think you've come to the right place. What Mark and Brant offer here is the key to discovering that extra something. It's what Mark was missing before he began to win Ironmans, and it could be what you're missing to realize your most authentic—fittest—self. If you do just one thing differently this week based on a single idea given, you will notice a change for the better and want to keep going.

Even though I've worked with many leaders and teachers throughout the years, I was both surprised and delighted with all their fresh material, unambiguous insights, and innovative exercises. On the one hand, it's deep but on the other it's practical and the manner in which Mark and Brant convey their knowledge and recommendations makes it easy for the reader to implement. It's one of the few books I've read that puts the undeniable mind-body connection into brilliant context and engaging terms, presenting exercises to fortify that fiercely rooted bond.

You will discover fresh new angles about "fitness" and lessons for developing a new habit in every chapter, some that will boost your emotional side and others that will help you to raise your physical health quotient. Try them all. I love how they start the book with a short questionnaire unlike any other that will get your engines running. You will quickly see just where you stand on their fitness meter. (Don't panic, there are no questions about blood pressure or how fast you can run a mile!) Many of the questions, and likely your answers, will get you thinking as you identify sources of stress in your life, ascertain how you feel about various aspects of yourself, and pinpoint where you could be going wrong in your quest for a better, more fulfilling existence.

Consider this the ultimate guide to complete well-being—an instructive book on how to reach your highest level of health and contentment through small, focused changes. It features nine keys that virtually everyone would do well to abide by. Of all the concepts and subjects Brant and Mark cover here, from goal-setting to tackling or managing stress, fear, anger, and jealousy, I think you'll find their attention to the power of nature (and how you can use it to strengthen your soul) to be exceptionally penetrative and thought-provoking. You don't hear many teachers talk about nature like Brant and Mark do. They will show you how to reconnect with the natural world and literally use its inherent strength to help you achieve more. No hocus-pocus in the least. You are likely to gain a set of tools you never thought to acquire before. For instance, have you ever wanted a proven way to literally turn off (or at least redirect) your mind when it starts rattling negative self-talk? Or a straightforward guide to conditioning both your body *and* your psyche? How about permission and tips to honoring yourself—to beating boredom and discovering inspiration *within yourself*? It's all in here. Don't let the fact this book lands in the health and fitness section prevent you from digesting every single page. It belongs on *every* bookshelf. The heart of this message applies to anyone looking to achieve personal greatness, pure and simple.

I trust you will share my passion for Mark and Brant's book and message. They are truly remarkable people from the inside out. Egoless. Authentic. Insightful far beyond the traditional classroom. As will become wonderfully clear to you, these two teachers carry a set of skills and knowledge unlike any others, and you will feel compelled to implement them into your life right away. Remember, no work equals no results. This roadmap will help make that work seem effortless, yet the rewards are limitless.

Contents

Welcome to a
New Approach to Life

*Having health of both body and spirit is what makes us
whole, happy people who feel good about life and can do
something as amazing as winning an Ironman . . .*

Imagine having a connection between your physical body and that inner, intangible part of you called the "soul" that is so powerful that you can do just about anything. Accomplish more at work. Lose unwanted weight. Gain vibrant health and more energy. Sleep like a baby at night. Have more satisfying relationships. Experience greater fulfillment in all that you do. Get into the best shape of your life. That is exactly what this book is going to help you to achieve, that and so much more. Sounds like a tall order, but not when you learn the elements to the Fit Soul, Fit Body Program.

Today, many of us have lost touch with our physicality, resulting in an epidemic of disease and disability due to our modern lifestyle. Obesity rates have soared in the United States, with estimates putting up to 65 percent of us in the overweight category. We have fallen to twenty-fourth on the worldwide list of longevity, when compared to other developed nations. In fact, some health professionals have suggested that today's generation of kids—about a third of whom are overweight or obese—may be the first who will live shorter lives than their parents. More and more children are also less healthy, showing increases in type 2 diabetes and heart disease, illnesses traditionally associated with adults. And among adults, only 10 percent of those who commit to exercising with their post–New Year's resolution will stick to it beyond three months.

But you have probably already been clued in to this current state of affairs from the media and recent news reports. More important to you now is how *you* can make a transformation in your own life through doable, small shifts in your lifestyle, and see measurable results.

Even if you regularly work out and maintain a healthy lifestyle, you may notice that there is still something missing that keeps you from feeling completely satisfied with your achievements. Have you experienced this? Maybe you are having difficulties staying inspired at work, feeling refreshed in the morning, or getting excited about planning for the future. These plateaus and stalls can end up causing self-doubt, low self-esteem, and even fear, all of which bring about one of the most difficult hurdles we all face: lack of motivation. Maybe you are bored with your workout regimen, you can't finish that 10k you've been training for, or you've started gaining weight despite your workouts and attention to your diet. Or perhaps you haven't been physically active in a while and deep down you know you need to get moving again. Considering the stresses that exist in our modern world, the last thing we need is for our lifestyle choices to contribute to our unhappiness.

Vibrant Health for Everyone

Starting in these first few pages, let's begin to see the word "fitness" in a whole new light. Fitness is for everyone because **today's health crisis is more than physical—it is also spiritual**. Try to avoid restricting this word to refer only to muscles, cardiovascular health, and the ability to, say, run a marathon. Being fit is not just for elite athletes, or even the people who regularly work out. When we say "Fit Soul, Fit Body," we are referring to two intertwining elements that must be in full force in order to attain and realize vibrant health. Not only are our physical markers of good health ("Fit Body") lagging, but so are the ones that measure our emotional health ("Fit Soul"). Seventy-six percent of us say we experience a notable amount of stress in our lives, which can lead to anxiety, a reduced sense of well-being, sleep deprivation, and a feeling that the world is something to be feared rather than revered. We lose sight of our goals and dreams, and have no idea how to get to where we want to be. As a nation, per person, we take more antidepressants than any of our Western-world counterparts.

Uncertainty and stress are not new to human beings. Our ancient ancestors had their share of challenges to staying alive in a world filled with wild animals and unpredictable food supplies. What is different nowadays is that we do not have a spiritual connection to life that infuses us with trust and the confidence that every-thing will work out in the end. We no longer tap in to the regenerative power in our environment. And it's easy to see why: Open landscapes are now city blocks, sunrises and sunsets take place while we are stuck in the confines of an office, and time spent soaking in nature's beauty has been replaced with calendars packed with meetings or endless hours online.

Countless fitness and self-help books address the crises of body and mind that so many of us experience today. And while these books are more popular than ever, none of them—and none of the gym memberships, exercise classes, or diet pills—are solving our problems. The reason these methods fail is that they treat the body and soul separately, instead of as two parts of one unified whole. The only way to improve our overall health is to tune in to the health of our emotions and spirit as we also tune in to our physicality. This doesn't just help us drop ten pounds or get into tip-top shape, it also creates a feeling of balance and connection to the world around us.

This connection between body and soul has been all but lost in the modern world. We have become like a phone that is not plugged in to the wall—the greatest message could be waiting but you will never hear it until you plug the phone back in. The same holds true for the signals our body and our environment are continuously giving us about how to build our physical, emotional, and spiritual health. When our souls get disconnected from our outer environment we can become lonely, depressed, even angry.

Most of us are too wound up, overworked, and tired to stop and listen. If we did, we would rediscover how to live a healthy life filled with lasting joy, happiness, and contentment. This book will be your roadmap to the ultimate Fit Soul, Fit Body, with tips and exercises to improve diet, fitness, and strength, and to find a renewed connection to the environment and natural world. Regardless of your individual goals, the ideas outlined in this book will help you to optimize every aspect of your life, from how you think to the actions you take to get whatever you want out of life. Best of all, the principles you will learn are timeless, and the longer you practice them, the more you will achieve and the more accomplished you will feel.

In This Book

Your Fit Body goals can be simple (losing weight, getting faster) or challenging (winning an Ironman). Your Fit Soul vision can also be small (feeling happy) to large (changing old patterns that have held you back for years). The program will work on all of these levels of desired change. We will follow guidelines taken from shamanic and indigenous teachings, which have been used for thousands of years to bring health and happiness. Shamanism originates from the universal relationship with the earth that all people have. We will bring you back to these simple yet profound guidelines, which can help you make significant and sustainable changes in both your body and your soul.

While this book does keep a focus on physical fitness—after all, we don't believe you can be physically unfit and emotionally fulfilled at the same time—you don't have to be a competitive athlete or workout warrior to benefit from the inspirational keys we share. And you don't have to be an outdoor enthusiast to recognize the importance of cultivating a relationship with nature as an antidote to the toll the modern world can take on us all. Regardless of your goals, drawing energy from the earth can help you increase strength, sharpen focus, relieve stress, and eradicate self-doubt.

You'll have the opportunity to gauge your overall wellness in the very first chapter of this book with a quiz. This brief test will also help you identify your strength and weaknesses so you can maximize the ideas shared in the book. Chapters 1 through 6 will cover the secrets to achieving a Fit Soul and a Fit Body, including nine simple keys that encapsulate the main message points and which you can apply to your own life starting today. A large part of the content in Chapters 1 through 4 will focus on the Fit Soul component. It helps to learn the Fit Soul exercises before undertaking the more specific Fit Body recommendations in Chapter 5, where you'll build your own personal conditioning program, and Chapter 6, which is devoted to nutritional strategies that you can tailor to your personal needs and fitness plans. You will also be given tools to connect with eating in a way that allows this simple act to become something spiritual, making food medicine for a healthy body and soul. Because the absence of a Fit Soul makes it so difficult, if not impossible, to achieve a truly Fit Body, we believe it's essential to start with that part of the program. The elements of Fit Soul give you a foundation from which to optimize your Fit Body. And in all, both sides—the Fit Soul and the Fit Body—ultimately work hand in hand to bring out the very best in yourself—physically, emotionally, mentally, and spiritually.

Sooner than you think, you will be embracing a new—and better—you. We will address the major impediments to attaining vibrant health, from boredom and burn-out to negative emotions like fear, jealousy, and anger. In addition to helping clarify what might be keeping you from experiencing fulfillment, we will offer a host of tried and true practical strategies to overcome obstacles and initiate positive outcomes. Finally, in Chapters 7 and 8 you'll find additional techniques to help reinforce and fortify the nine keys in your life, plus ideas on troubleshooting your way through setbacks while you continue to live by the tenets of Fit Soul, Fit Body.

Sprinkled throughout the book will be our own personal stories, which are meant to inspire and entertain you while at the same time demonstrate the power of these teachings. The stories of Mark's journey as a competitive triathlete in particular serve to show you how these techniques and lessons can come into play during the most challenging of events. If they can help you win Ironman championships, imagine what they can do in your day-to-day life, far from a traditional racecourse. Whatever your dreams and goals may be, these keys will help you to get "unstuck," to push past whatever is holding you back physically, mentally, and emotionally, and to discover the limitless achievements that await you.

To supplement your experience in this book, we invite you to log on to our Web site at www.fitsoulfitbody.com and access resources and further information and tools that can help you in your journey. You'll find some of the more technical tips and nutritional insights on our Web site, which is ideal for those who choose to apply this program to any rigorous event. By the time you reach the end of this book, you will be poised to discover a life without limits. And you will have already commenced a new approach to life.

Note to the reader: At times we will fall into storytelling mode, using the personal "I." It will either be Brant's or Mark's voice, and you will know which is which. Any first-person story about competing in the Ironman will be Mark speaking, and you'll hear Mark in most of the chapter openings. The stories of his experiences and the trials of his competitive spirit say a lot about how this program came to be, and how it can change you, too. Any story relating the Huichol tradition or Don José Matsuwa, who was Brant's mentor and became his adopted Huichol grandfather and close companion, will be Brant speaking.

Chapter One

A Fit Body's Secret Ingredient: A Fit Soul

You can only do so much with the body, and so much more with the mind . . .

What does it mean to be fit? How fit can a person be? How fit are *you* right now? By the end of this chapter you're going to know the answers to these questions. To begin to understand exactly what we mean by having a Fit Body, let's cast back to the year 1989. There is no better way to illustrate the unlimited power of a Fit Soul within the confines of the physical body than to tell the story of Mark's attempt to win the Ironman that year.

Fifty-Eight Seconds and a Soul, as Told by Mark

When I began my career as a professional triathlete in 1982, I judged my success in terms of the minutes and seconds I could shave off my competitive times. For the first six years of my career, I focused on the fitness of my body, and I won plenty of races, but I always fell short of my goal—the Ironman World Championship. It wasn't until I met Brant Secunda and learned how to think of fitness in broader terms—in terms of my spirit and emotions—that I was able to become the champion I aspired to be and find the strength of spirit I had been seeking.

7

The Ironman takes a simple idea and makes it complex: To achieve victory all you have to do is go faster than everyone else. But this one-day journey through the lava at Kona, on the Big Island of Hawaii, is a test like no other. It's an exhaustive trial of body and soul that starts with a 2.4-mile open-ocean swim. This is followed immediately by 112 miles of cycling through relentless, hot trade winds along the dry, desolate, lava-strewn west side of the Big Island. The race concludes with a marathon—26.2 miles of running in temperatures that are in the high nineties.

My first six years racing at the Ironman varied from moderately disappointing to outright disastrous. Flat tires, flat legs, and internal bleeding all kept me from achieving my dream of becoming the champion of that great event. I humbly accepted six straight defeats at the Ironman, always delaying my dream of winning for one more year. After so many failed attempts, my patience and confidence were failing. By 1989, seven years into my career as a triathlete, I was questioning whether I should just give up on my dream of winning the Ironman altogether.

I certainly had the desire to win. But desire has a shelf life of about three hours under the intense sun and wind of Hawaii, and it provides little insulation from the parts of you that are fearful or uncertain. When exhaustion and self-doubt overcame me, my motivation would deteriorate to the point that I just wanted to give up. I began to realize that it wasn't a failure of my body that was keeping me from winning; it was a failure of my mind. I needed more than just a Fit *Body*—I needed a Fit *Soul*. But at the time, I had no idea what that was or how to develop it.

In 1989 I committed myself to making one final attempt at the race I had envisioned but had been unable to achieve. My seventh (and what I thought would be my final) Ironman started as all the others did. I felt good and held a decent position through the swim and bike sections. But I was still burdened by my past failures. My nemesis was the world record holder for the Ironman, a man named Dave Scott, who by 1989 had amassed a total of six Ironman titles.

Dave and I raced the first two legs of the event—swimming and cycling—as we had every other year, always keeping within striking distance of each other. Then the run came. We were side by side, but he was definitely the stronger of the two of us. Dave set a pace that was beyond anything I thought was humanly possible; by keeping up with him, we were both on track to break his three-year-old record. By the halfway point in the marathon, the rest of the field had melted away, leaving me the last man with a chance to break Dave's winning streak.

Dave shifted gears, upping the pace to a six-minute mile. I responded, but barely. My reserves were reaching their limit. As Dave held his surge, I had just enough energy to entertain a few passing thoughts, none of which were the kind that might help me win the race. *This is too much. My legs are killing me. Dave is too strong. He's going to win again. I'll never win this ridiculous race. If I let him go, even an inch, he's won. I can't do it. I'm such a loser.* Luckily, only a few more moments would pass before a transformation took place which—at the time—defied my sense of reason.

Dave's relentless pace became so difficult to match that even the negative thoughts were impossible to conjure up. All my energy was channeled into holding on to what meager hope I had of keeping my Ironman dream alive. Then my mind went quiet, and suddenly I caught sight of something hovering just above the lava to my right. It was a man, someone I'd seen before.

A week before this Ironman day, I had been mindlessly flipping through a magazine that I had no real interest in reading. Near the front was an advertisement that caught my eye, featuring a picture of two men—an old Huichol man from Mexico named Don José Matsuwa, and his adopted grandson, Brant Secunda. Both men were shamans, and they were going to be hosting a workshop about this tradition as it is practiced by the Huichols. In the photograph, Brant looked both gentle and powerful. There was a peace in his face that I had never seen before. Don José was dressed in traditional Huichol clothing: a white, loose-fitting costume embroidered with vibrant designs, and a colorful straw hat. He had a smile that seemed to be saying, "I am happy just to be alive."

During the race, in that moment of internal silence, I saw Don José again, and his calm, reassuring smile. Was he real or was I dreaming? I snapped my head to the right, but he was gone. So I turned back and focused on the road of crushed lava that was passing beneath my feet. I told myself to just put one foot in front of the other—no matter what. Once more my mind went quiet. And there again was Don José, smiling with gratitude for life, and I could feel energy coming from him.

The best race Ironman had ever seen was now entering its seventh hour, and race officials on mopeds and a throng of well-wishers on bicycles crowded the road ahead of Dave and me. The ABC camera van directly in front of us was shooting this moment of uncertainty. The tension of the close competition gripped everyone present. Not a word was uttered. The only sound was the squishing of four sweat-soaked shoes as they came down on the pavement, over and over. Everyone was focused solely on the unfolding race. But me? I was having visions of one of the greatest shamans of modern times.

There were still thirteen miles left to this grueling race. Dave was continuing his otherworldly surge to my left, but something inside me had changed. Instead of the crushing weight of my impending defeat, I was now incredibly thankful to still be racing side by side with the best triathlete in the world. I looked around at the lava that had caused me so many struggles, and I felt such gratitude to be running over one of the natural wonders of the world, the Big Island. I no longer needed to win to feel good. Being a part of the race was enough.

Dave kept upping the pace. It was clear that what I thought was a brief surge was actually a steady, unrelenting acceleration. We both knew at mile 24.5, with less than two miles to go in the race, that there would be one last arduous climb before descending to the finish line and the winner's tape. Both of us were planning to use this hill as the breaking point. There was one last aid station at the bottom of this critical hill. I suspected that Dave's idea was to grab a final cup of water and then make his decisive play for victory.

Trump.

I made my move as we went through the station, forgoing fuel in the hope that turning up the pace would be enough to pull ahead. Just as Dave turned to grab his final glass from an aid station volunteer, I sprinted (as best as I could at the end of an Ironman). By the time Dave turned back, I had opened up a gap of several feet.

Now it was his turn to respond. He tried ferociously, but ultimately he couldn't.

My margin of victory over Dave was one of the smallest in Ironman history—fifty-eight seconds. Dave beat his world-record time by more than fifteen minutes. I bettered my previous best by nearly twenty-five minutes. That day marked the end of a long journey at Kona. It also signaled the beginning of another.

Shaping a Fit Soul to Achieve a Fit Body

After the race, I told my friends about my vision of Don José. I wasn't surprised they thought the physical and emotional exhaustion of the day had clouded my thinking. I would have thought the same thing myself before this incredible experience. Others tried to rationalize and explain away my experience, but to me it seemed like the most natural thing that could have happened.

From the outside it looked like the significance of that day was winning after so many defeats. But vastly more important was experiencing for the first time my own connection of body and soul. Something deeper and more enduring than the fleeting thrill of victory had touched me. The thirst for winning was quenched, but another, stronger one had replaced it and called me to begin studying with Brant. By the next year I had started a journey that continues to this day: learning from this great teacher about a wondrous way of life that weaves good health into pursuits of both my soul and my body.

His teachings, practices, and tools for transformation, many of which are in this book, helped me to change pain into joy, inner struggle into gratitude, impatience and fear into calm and courage . . . all things that support reaching one's goals, whether they are about racing, fitness, personal change, or simply having a more positive outlook on life. He helped me move from having low self-esteem to trusting in life. He enabled me to change a sense of hopelessness into a clarity of purpose. He gave me the tools to hold on and keep going, even when life's most devastating setbacks were thrown my way. Brant taught me how to quiet my Western mind, which was always busy analyzing and judging every moment of life as good or bad, a mind that more often than not sabotaged my chances for success, something that became key to excelling in the unpredictable world of Ironman racing. He opened my heart so that the real answers and solutions to life's dilemmas could be heard. And these were the easy things!

Perhaps the toughest changes Brant has helped me to make, and certainly some of the most profound, have been the ones that taught me about humility and the freedom one can experience through it. There was very little that was glamorous about the training it took to be a champion. But with Brant's help I was able to humbly surrender to that reality. Then, instead of resisting my training, I was free and motivated to do the workouts over and over that built the fitness my dreams were asking for.

His tools of transformation have given me the strength to face truth, which is often easier to push away than to accept and deal with. He helped me to experience the freedom that envelops one's life when truth is indeed embraced. He has given me hope where there was none before, the vision to see change as possible, and the life force and energy to live what the great dreams of my life are calling for.

Brant is both a teacher and a healer. After years during which pregnancy looked impossible, he brought about the life of my son through an incredible fertility healing. He has healed everything in my physical body, from a broken collarbone and knees that were weakening to cancer from so many hours spent in the sun. In the years between my first victory in 1989 and my sixth in 1995, Brant put me back together over and over when the diagnosis of traditional Western doctors was telling me to quit. He silenced those who said I would never even be able to start the race, let alone win it!

I asked for his help to be prepared and ready for the toughest single-day endurance event of our time. This was a tall order, but one that Brant was able to help me achieve year after year. Deceptively simple on the surface, the practices he had me do over and over had profound results. Some of these key practices are in this book, ready to be embraced by you in your life when faced with your personal Ironman. Just living the simple wisdom that Brant spoke year after year can change your life dramatically. "Be steady" were his words to help me navigate life's challenges without being thrown off course. "Laughter is medicine for the soul" was his credo that lightened my toughest trials and kept them in perspective. Over and over he would tell me to "Be fearless in the face of your fears"— eight simple words that erased thoughts of quitting and fortified my soul with resolve and hope. Without Brant my stories of Ironman racing would not speak of victory, but only defeat. Without his teaching and guidance, I would be just another athlete who pushed his body to the limit only to find out at the end of his career that success is really a matter of heart and soul. But because of him my life has purpose, hope, and happiness . . . three qualities that will breathe life and positive energy into any endeavor, and that can fuel your personal journey of having a Fit Soul and a Fit Body.

Understand the Crisis of Body and Mind

If you're like most people, you define fitness solely in terms of your body and your physical capabilities—how big your muscles are, how fast you can run, how many stairs you can climb without feeling winded, or how much you weigh. As we mentioned in the Introduction, we want to give you a different model of health and fitness, one that addresses not only your body, but also the human being that is housed inside. Working out will certainly give you a wonderful outer appearance. But if the person you are behind the chiseled body with six-pack abs does not experience inherent happiness with life, the picture will not be complete. Just look at the number of professional athletes who have bodies of steel but turn to drugs and bad behavior hoping to find the things they are missing—happiness, fulfillment, inner peace.

We want to give you both, a Fit Soul and a Fit Body. While at first the concept of having a fit soul may seem strange, keep in mind that most people already link many aspects of their emotional and spiritual feelings to the state of their fitness. Who among us hasn't hoped that transforming our physical self would be a cure for a negative self-image—that losing fifty pounds, dropping three clothes sizes, or running a faster mile would resolve feelings of low self-esteem, fear, anger, depression, or jealousy? But even when traditional fitness goals are achieved, what most people quickly realize is that you can change your body and still not be happy or fulfilled. The numbers may be what you wanted, but the feeling is not. You hit a barrier. Then your motivation to work out or diet wanes because you don't feel like you thought you would.

The reason we fall short of our goals so often is that exercise is part, but not all, of the answer. True health and happiness is about developing a sustainable lifestyle where you not only achieve long-term physical health, but also long-term emotional and spiritual health. This is what we call having both a Fit Soul and a Fit Body.

What Is a Soul?

Whatever religion you practice—or don't—the concept of a soul is universal. Your soul is the sum of all you have experienced in life as well as your perception of those experiences, both good and bad. It's the joy and the sadness, the happiness and the pain. It's the place of peace that can experience the world as a wonder and your life as a magical event going on in it. Your soul is the resolve that gets you through tough times and forgives you when you cannot.

Your soul is who you inherently are, and is a part of your self that is connected to all of creation. It is dynamic, not static. Its gauge changes depending on the choices you make and the actions you take. A Fit Soul is one whose meter is usually pointed in a positive direction. It has strength and energy for real purpose in life and is the counterweight that pulls you up when life seems to be conspiring to draw you down. A Fit Soul is filled with laughter, joy, and pure happiness. It moves through the tough times always searching for the answers to life's quests. A Fit Soul is filled with light. It sparkles in the presence of others as well as in the silence of one's own solitude.

What Shamanism Can Teach Us

Your soul naturally yearns to be in sync with your body. Having true health starts by recognizing that a Fit Soul and a Fit Body are integrated elements of real vitality and well-being. The model we will use for developing this integrated approach to life comes from the

Huichols, who are an indigenous culture living in central Mexico. For a Huichol, the health of the body and spirit is an integral part of daily life, a result of living in cooperation with family, friends, and nature. Contrast the Huichol outlook to that of Western sports and Western culture, which are based on competition, on seeing oneself as a rival against others.

Shamanism is a system of healing and living in harmony with the spirit of nature. It adheres to the belief that everything is alive and has a spirit—trees, flowers, mountains, lakes, rivers, and of course animals. Huichol shamanism, like the shamanism of many indigenous cultures, is based on cooperation, on seeing oneself as a collaborator with all life. In this book, you will learn how to go beyond your traditional understanding of competition and your own physical, emotional, mental, and even spiritual limitations. By finding your place in the world and feeling at home in it, you will not only be more successful in your fitness pursuits, but will also be able to live with greater joy and satisfaction.

Living in the Sierra Madre mountains, the Huichols are known as a nation of shamans. They have no history of war, and today they consist of about 30,000 people. They are said to be the last tribe in North America to have maintained their pre-Columbian traditions. At one point in time, almost half of the population were healers, indigenous doctors, and ceremonial leaders. Huichol cosmology regarding good health is simultaneously simple and quite profound. They believe that our spirit is connected to our heart, and, of course, our heart is in our body. The Huichols maintain that by simply walking on the earth we can heal our body, and that through thinking good thoughts—connecting to the sunrise, the sunset, other humans, and the world around us—we naturally heal our soul. The Huichols believe that the soul, our higher self that is connected to all life, is not just an abstract concept. They say good health happens through a union of two important aspects all human beings have— the body and soul.

We will be sharing the elements of Huichol life that are useful for achieving a strong body and a healthy soul. These elements apply to everyone, no matter where you live on this magnificent planet. All of us are indeed brothers and sisters united just by living on the earth.

It's our common past, not our current differences, that we will use to develop a way of living that can bring complete well-being into our own lives.

Awakening to a Shaman's World, As Told by Brant

Before I met the Huichols the connection of body and soul was something I had never heard of. But through my education with them, I saw how this connection is expressed in every aspect of their existence. The Huichol idea of fitness does not include Western sports or gym workouts. Their daily activities include chopping and carrying firewood and growing the five beautiful colors of corn. This is physically demanding work that requires strength of the body. And for the Huichols, this is also profoundly spiritual work. We can use their example to make our bodies strong and fit while at the same time using the natural environment to heal our souls.

My journey to Mexico to visit the Huichols began after I graduated from high school and had traveled around the USA. I had heard stories of these somewhat mysterious and legendary people living high up in the mountains of central Mexico who were celebrated for their visionary artwork and traditional ceremonial lifestyle, and I wanted to see them for myself. I was ready for an adventure and had been yearning to travel far from the confines of my American home life in New Jersey. So I said good-bye to my parents, who wished me well and who understood my need to travel at this point in my life. None of us knew where my journey would take me, nor did any of us realize that this would mark the start of my life as a Huichol.

I traveled through Mexico by bus. This was a time of many firsts for me. I had never seen a farm or vegetables growing until my journey across the country; at a stop in Colorado, I mistook the sounds of crickets for a rattlesnake and nearly scared myself to death. Eventually I arrived in Ixtlan, a small town nestled in the Sierra Madre mountains. This mountain range is also known as the "Huichol Sierra," since only Huichol people are permitted to live in and pass through this area. Because these mountains are incredibly rugged and inaccessible, the Huichols have been able to live isolated from the modern world, practicing their age-old traditions of shamanism, for thousands of years.

My journey into this rugged land was far from a holiday. It started with a treacherous prop-plane ride through jutting peaks and dipping valleys. After that I still had a five-day hike to find the village of a Huichol schoolteacher who had given me a letter of invitation to journey into this sacred land. I walked, feeling a slight wind in my face breathing life into me that I didn't know I needed. I had two pineapples and a canteen of water. As you can imagine, all this was gone in the opening hours of my hike. I continued on anyway, and on the third day of my trek I became completely lost and disoriented. This was certainly not New York with a street sign at every corner. I was hopelessly lost in a maze of tiny deer trails. I knew I was suffering from dehydration and sun exposure. I began to panic. The worst thought to me was that no one would even know what had happened to me. It would have helped my attitude if I could have just laughed a little at my predicament, but I was too afraid. I knew I was dying.

I stopped and took out a pen and paper and wrote my parents a letter, hoping that if I didn't make it, someone would find the note and give it to them. I would like to say I faced my death like a spiritual warrior, but the reality was that I was facing it like a spiritual crybaby. Tearful and cynical that no one was there to rescue me, I passed out.

I don't know how long I was unconscious, but suddenly I was awakened and saw Indians standing over me, sprinkling water onto my face, nudging me ever so carefully, telling me to wake up and stop acting like a drunkard. One of the men said that his father, Don Juan (not the one of Castaneda fame), the old shaman of their village, had had a dream about me two days prior and that they had been sent out to bring me back to their village.

I was dumbfounded that someone I had never met could dream I was in trouble, and I could only mumble. One of the men handed me a gourd filled with delicious water, which I eagerly consumed. The group of Huichols then led me back to their village, laughing and talking almost continuously among themselves. Because we all spoke Spanish, there were no barriers, and eventually I would learn how to speak their native Huichol language, too. When we arrived at the village, the shaman told me we would offer prayers of thankfulness to the four directions. This was the beginning of my giving thanks and learning to make myself humble. Prayer allows you to open your heart and be free; it empowers you. The Huichols say it takes nine years to learn how to pray. Just as a surgeon takes many years to perfect his or her craft, the art of prayer is perfected for anyone trying over time, and this was my beginning. I was praying from my heart and giving thanks. Prayer gives you a reason for living, and I was definitely happy that I was alive. I had not been brought up with any specific religion, and I found myself embracing this opportunity to grow a deeper, more spiritual side of myself.

I was later taken to the village of Don José Matsuwa, an exceptionally powerful and wise elder of the Huichol tribe, who offered to take me as his apprentice and to adopt me as his grandson. As part of my arduous shamanic education, Don José and I walked throughout the Huichol Sierra to many beautiful and sacred places of power. We journeyed to the mountain where the sun was born in a windblown desert land many miles from the Huichol Sierra. We grew corn, gathered firewood, and I participated, along with Don José and other members of the tribe, in many ceremonies to celebrate and honor the four seasons.

Throughout the next twelve years, Mexico became my main home away from home, as I ended up doing an apprenticeship with Don José that would change the course and significance of my life forever. He taught me that we could enjoy even the most difficult things in life and find happiness in the process of learning and changing. The Huichol model for life does not emphasize thinking and analyzing as much as we do in the modern world, but rather they practice just being present in the moment—every moment. Slowly but surely, a magical transformation began. I was no longer that brash city kid looking for adventure. My training was indeed difficult, but also joyful. As a Huichol I learned to live through my heart, experiencing the world around me through the medium of feeling.

Nurtured and prodded by the fierce yet immensely loving tutelage of Don José, my body and spirit, which for so long had barely coexisted with one another, were becoming one whole entity. To see with your heart as well as your eyes is transformational. To hear with your heart as well as your ears is also transformational. My body breathed in the different aromas surrounding me. My ears listened to the wind whistling across the dense mountain foliage. My eyes became aware of the beauty of the corn growing in the fields, the spectacular sunrises and sunsets, and the thousands of stars overhead. These were all impressions from nature that changed my soul. This was all so very different from my experience growing up in a North American city.

Don José was not only a great spiritual leader, but he was also a man of great physical strength. He stood just over five feet tall, but he could carry 100 pounds of firewood on his back straight up a mountain that I could barely walk up empty-handed. His life was an example that anything is possible—physically, mentally, and spiritually.

The Huichols show us that a simple way of being can transform our life and help us to accomplish many things, such as becoming fit and getting in touch with our souls. Fit Soul, Fit Body naturally brings together cohesive ingredients that enhance our ability to be healthy, happy, and strong. It is a natural health program and a way to living in balance on the earth.

When I met Mark and we began working together, it became evident that there are many ways to bring together the worlds of sport and spirit. Just as Mark brought together swimming, biking, and running great distances in the incredible Ironman races, I recognized that the bridge to the Huichol way of being is connected to the diverse elements of body and soul, earth and sky. The Huichols walk many miles on the earth, praying and hoping for a positive outcome. It was not always assured that they would be able to finish a long pilgrimage or journey. They had to work for it, just as Mark had to work hard to finish his races and bring completion to his life. I was able to teach Mark that nothing is impossible and that our efforts are empowered by our thoughts and attitudes in life.

A Huichol model for good health and fitness goes beyond having just a strong body. I used this perspective to inspire Mark with Huichol stories of creation, and through my apprenticeship with Don José, led him through many exercises that gave him both physical power and emotional inspiration. We walked on the earth, danced on the earth, prayed at the edge of oceans, lakes, rivers. All of this combined to help make Mark a world-class athlete. Amazing personal transformations like this are possible for virtually everyone.

Find Your Own Fifty-Eight Seconds

If you only take away one message from this book, let it be this: **Having strength of body *and* soul is the secret to living a full life**. A strong body makes just about everything you do a little easier. A strong soul allows you to find peace in the midst of calamity. Our definition of "strength," however, may be different from the popular understanding of it. Strength does not necessarily imply having monstrous muscles that are the envy of every bodybuilder. Nor does it mean having a will of steel that plows through life like a bulldozer. Of course, strong muscles and a sound resolve have their place. But the type of strength that we will help you develop also has resiliency. Don José and Mark had incredible physical strength without big, bulky, muscle-bound bodies.

Each living thing on this planet reflects this fine balance between strength and flexibility. Trees grow tall as they strengthen themselves with the energy of the sun, earth, water, and air. They also bend and sway in the wind without breaking. Good health depends upon this idea. Your ability to "sway in the wind"—to respond to life's challenges, changes, joys, and stresses—without breaking requires resiliency of both body and soul.

These strengths are what enable us as human beings to feel at home in any situation we come across. Everything from getting in and out of bed to the most demanding physical sports benefit from developing resilient strength. Too much strength and you become rigid. Too little, and a back can get thrown out or a muscle pulled. Your soul is the same. A strong soul sways under the pressure of life's challenges but doesn't break. Those who thrive are able to find peace and keep a clear spirit when tested by life.

The principles of Fit Soul, Fit Body work in natural ways to bring about positive changes in your health and your life. Our advice and exercises will help you to transform the negative emotions we all have in common (self-doubt, fear, anger, jealousy) into positive ones we all yearn for (joy, happiness, peace). The main tenets explored in this book are universal—they apply to everyone, whether you want to boost your health, be a world-class athlete, or simply enhance the quality of your life. And even if you don't aspire to become an athlete, just knowing you have the tools to do so will work in other areas of your life. In other words, you'll find your own fifty-eight-second lead in whatever it is that you want to do exceptionally well.

Test Your Wellness

It helps to have a general idea of where your overall health in mind, body, and spirit stands today so you can maximize your journey forward and identify where you could be paying closer attention. Following is a brief quiz we've put together to help you gauge your level of wellness—from the inside out. It's unlike other health tests you may have taken because we won't ask you about your cholesterol level or number on the scale. Be honest with yourself as you answer these questions. You don't have to share your responses with anyone. We encourage you to revisit this quiz whenever you want, to see if any of your answers have changed for the better. You can always come back to this quiz as a way of checking in with yourself and see how you're doing.

1) I am generally:
   - ☐ Happy and fulfilled (3 points)
   - ☐ Somewhat happy but searching for something (1 point)
   - ☐ Depressed and emotionally out of control (0 points)

2) I experience stress:
   - ☐ Only occasionally (2 points)
   - ☐ More often than I'd like to admit (1 point)
   - ☐ Chronically; it's never-ending (0 points)

3) When faced with stress, I:
   - ☐ Use strategies that help me navigate through successfully (3 points)
   - ☐ Am moderately able to deal with it (1 point)
   - ☐ Completely lose it. Leave me alone! (0 points)

4) I spend time with a community of friends:
   □ One or more days a week—no matter what (3 points)
   □ One day a month—maybe, if I can fit it in (2 points)
   □ Almost never; who has time for that? (0 points)

5) I spend:
   □ Every day in nature (3 points)
   □ One day a week in nature (2 points)
   □ One day a month in nature (1 point)
   □ Virtually no time in nature (0 points)

6) I watch a sunrise or sunset:
   □ Once a week (3 points)
   □ A few times a month (2 points)
   □ Once in a while (1 points)
   □ Almost never (0 points)

7) I have negative qualities such as jealousy and fear that I would like to change.
   □ Disagree. I am mostly positive (3 points)
   □ Somewhat agree (1 point)
   □ Strongly agree (0 points)

8) I feel my spiritual health is:
   □ Of equal importance to my physical health (3 points)
   □ Of greater importance than my physical health (1 point)
   □ Of less importance than my physical health (0 points)

9) I exercise:
   □ Never (0 points)
   □ 1–2 hours per week (1 point)
   □ 3–4 hours per week (2 point)
   □ More than 4 hours per week (3 points)

10) I find exercise:
   □ Enjoyable (3 points)
   □ Tolerable (2 points)
   □ Worse than going to the dentist (0 points)

11) I usually:
- ☐ Push myself to the limit in workouts (2 points)
- ☐ Exercise at moderate levels (3 points)
- ☐ Rarely break a sweat (0 points)

12) I think I am able to make positive body composition changes.
- ☐ Strongly agree (3 points)
- ☐ Moderately agree (1 point)
- ☐ I find it tough to ever see myself changing (0 points)

13) I feel my weight:
- ☐ Is fairly ideal (3 points)
- ☐ Could use some modification (2 points)
- ☐ Cannot seem to stabilize (0 points)

14) I set clear goals for personal change.
- ☐ Strongly agree (3 points)
- ☐ Somewhat agree (2 points)
- ☐ I don't set goals (0 points)

15) When it comes to change, I generally:
- ☐ Follow through with my plan (3 points)
- ☐ Stumble, but then pick up where I left off (2 points)
- ☐ Feel like I am always starting over (0 points)

The higher your score, the healthier you are in mind, body, and spirit. The lower your score, the less fit you are overall and the more you will benefit from our teachings. If you scored less than ten points, you are a prime candidate for taking every principle in this book seriously and going at whatever pace you need to apply each key to your life. Bear in mind that it may take time for your body to respond to a shift in your lifestyle, however great or small. Give yourself a "breaking in" period. Some of these habits can eventually create new neuronal pathways in your body. That's right: the brain is not as hard-wired as we previously thought. The moment you decide to adapt these ideas to your life is the moment you begin to make physical, neurochemical, and hormonal changes in your body for the better—ones that will support your goal of bringing out your absolute best. Small changes add up and can have a big impact.

Virtually everyone can benefit from this program, including those who would say they lead healthy, happy lives, or who scored more than thirty points on the quiz. Other questions you may want to ask yourself (write down the answers in a journal) are:

- What do you do when faced with difficult situations?
- What do you do to solve them?
- What four negative qualities would you like to change?

Then look at your answers and see if you would like to change them. For example, if you face difficult situations with anger or resort to unhealthy habits like drinking too much, eating poorly, and avoiding exercise, then the keys in this book will help you develop fresh, healthy coping skills. If qualities like jealously, resentment, stress, and worry consume you, this program will help you to transform those self-defeating qualities into positive one for the soul.

Take note of the answers in the quiz that got you zero points. Let those be your focal points as you move forward. You may already be physically fit but lack that soulful fitness. Or maybe you feel grounded in your heart and soul, but need to give your physical fitness an overhaul. Remember that you've picked up this book for a reason. A little voice inside your head is telling you that it's time to make a change. Whatever that change may be, the Fit Soul, Fit Body Program will be your launching pad.

Expect Great Results

Discovering unprecedented health, balance, and well-being is not a mythological endeavor. When you incorporate the basic elements for a fit soul and body, you can realize tremendous results. This involves taking time to release negative qualities and adopt positive ones for the soul. It also involves exercise, diet, and strength training for the body. All of this happens when we are inspired and motivated to change, to improve our overall fitness and quality of life.

For a Huichol today, there is no separation between physical and spiritual health. For them, walking on the earth is both a physical effort (especially in the mountains where they live) and a chance to develop their spiritual connection with the earth. Growing corn requires a huge physical effort to prepare the hillsides for planting. It is also a chance to pray or ask for good crops, to ask that the rains come, and to be attuned to the four seasons.

Most of us in the modern world don't have cornfields to prepare, nor do we have wood and water to carry, nor do we take the time to absorb the power of nature. This is when we lose our physical health and become primed for one of the biggest challenges facing inhabitants of the modern world: stress. Because of this, we will begin your journey by helping you to lessen the impact of stress, as well as other negative emotions, which as you will see are often the core issues restricting one's inability to change both body and soul. After a firm grounding in a variety of Fit Soul techniques, we will start you on your way by helping you to create realistic goals and working with the principles needed for having a Fit Body in the modern world, which is more conducive to sitting than moving. As you learn the specifics of building a conditioning program and making optimal diet choices, we will help you to blend in those Fit Soul guidelines. The combination of all the exercises and ideas will help bring you back to the experiences that were designed to soothe our spirits and give us confidence in life and happiness to be a part of it. Special times of the day, like sunrise and sunset, will become your elixir of happiness. The four directions will become natural places for you to release negativity. The four elemental powers—earth, air, fire, and water—will be the spiritual cleansers which help you relieve stress and experience freedom.

Some of the transformations you experience from the Fit Body aspect of the program will be what you expect, such as increased strength, speed, and stamina. Best of all, everyone from top athletes to first timers will find that by using the Fit Body principles—and integrating the Fit Soul exercises—their goals will not only be achievable but also sustainable. As you focus on using the exercises and guidelines of both Fit Soul and Fit Body, you will also find that positive body composition changes take place, like weight loss and increased tone. In our program, these are benefits of developing overall wellness, and they will help you avoid the plateaus and unmet promises of programs designed solely around weight loss or improved physical appearance. One very important aspect of this will be a look at nutrition. Not everybody is going to need the same recommendations on how to eat for health. We will help you identify your specific body's needs and guide you along a progressive eating program that will bring you an optimal physical transformation.

There might also be some pleasant surprises along the way. For example, studies have shown that regular exercise increases many measurable features like memory, intelligence, reaction response time, and the ability to concentrate. In addition, aerobic exercise often produces a feeling of peaceful well-being, decreases and relieves the negative effects of stress, and improves a person's sense of self-esteem and self-confidence. Best of all, aerobic exercise can be something as simple and natural as walking.

Adopting the exercises needed to have a Fit Soul and Fit Body will help shift the core of who you are so that old patterns end and new ones begin. Low self-esteem, feeling isolated or alone, sensing your body's physical weakness, and being unmotivated will be transformed into universally positive qualities like joy, being inspired by life, feeling strong and agile, and having abundant energy to stay active and feel alive. The power of love will replace anger. Courage will transcend fear. Gratitude will overcome jealousy. Armed with the twin powers of Fit Soul, Fit Body, nearly any transformation you want will be possible.

Chapter Two
Conquer Stress

In the quiet of the heart, no stress can reside . . . only joy, power, and hope.

During the 1991 Ironman competition, I used a technique Brant taught me to win my third title. As I transitioned into the marathon portion of the competition, my mind began to race too. It was the kind of unfocused mental chatter that gets going and becomes extremely distracting. At the time, I was about five and a half hours into the event, and I found myself running behind a steely competitor named Cristián Bustos of Chile. His reputation as a strong endurance runner had made me fearful before the race. During the opening miles of the marathon, as I watched him pull ahead of me, the fear became severe and I took on defeated-type thoughts, like: *I can't keep up with him any longer. I don't know why I'm doing this stupid race. I won't win.* All the thoughts that can easily trick you into giving up sped through my brain.

Even when I caught up to him several miles later, the challenge was not yet over. He took one look over at me, upped his pace, and pulled away again, staying just in front of me, but not letting me run next to him. That was it. I couldn't take it any more. My mind went wild trying to convince me to drop out. Finally, I remembered the simple words that I had heard Brant say so many times: **"Be quiet. Quiet the mind. Pay attention to the beauty that surrounds you."**

It took some minutes, but I was finally able to do just that, to quiet my mind. I knew it was going to be impossible to come up with a positive thought at that moment, so it was better to have no thoughts at all. And in the instant that my mind went quiet, there was a subtle yet profound shift in the dynamic of the race.

I couldn't tell if I started to speed up or if Bustos began to slow down, but I could see that he was no longer pulling away from me. A mile later I was the one in control of the pace, and at the halfway point of this final leg of the Ironman, I pulled away with a surge that he could not answer. I then went on to win my third title. All from quieting the mind!

The Root of Many Evils

Quieting the mind is just one technique for removing the negative noise that can start streaming through your head in times of stress. We'll take you through an exercise to help you do this shortly. No doubt you've experienced mindless chatter at some point, even when you're not dashing to a finish line in a race. Not only does it divert your attention from the task at hand, but it further adds to your level of stress, which then has its own negative consequences on your body and spirit.

Of all the negative influences that can hold each of us back from having the spark we need to take action and affect positive change in our lives, the biggest one is stress. Trust in life and hope are good remedies for it, but can be tough to feel in a world where many only experience the stress. Just about everyone growing up today is affected by stress. The National Institute for Occupational Safety and Health found that stress causes a decreased willingness to take on new endeavors, can directly be blamed for up to 40 percent of job burnout, and will become **the number one occupational disease in this century**—causing more work days lost than any other factor. Stress is also linked to the top six causes of death in the United States: heart disease, cancer, lung ailments, accidents, cirrhosis of the liver, and suicide.

Stress can weaken your immune system, deplete energy, sap motivation, cause memory loss, and make it difficult to concentrate.

It disrupts sleep, which inhibits your ability to recover from a work-out or hard day at the office, and depletes the amount of energy needed for the next day's demands. As sleep deprivation accumu-lates, other areas of your life become affected, from relationships to work to the inspiration you feel for accomplishing your goals. Over time, stress, even at low levels, can lead to malaise and depression, both of which inhibit a positive outlook on life. Emotional and phys-ical stresses feed into each other to create a state that makes it nearly impossible to achieve long-term fitness for your body and your soul.

In ancient times and in indigenous cultures today, offsetting stress can be as simple as an afternoon siesta or gathering together to share in good-hearted laughter. We will draw from this simplicity to provide you with modern-world solutions to the six most common forms of stress in life—emotional, sleep deprivation induced, dietary, physical, chemical, and inflammation induced. This will be the first step toward being motivated and feeling inspired to have long-term health and well-being.

Kupuri = *Life Force*

One of the main goals in the world of the Huichols is to obtain life force and energy in our everyday life. *Kupuri* is the Huichol word for this powerful essence. Our goal is to obtain or gather kupuri from our environment and charge ourselves up with this natural life energy. One example is to go to a special place in nature or even sit under a tree and imagine the life force of this special place nurturing your soul. This is one simple way to conquer stress in our everyday life, no matter where we live. The world is a natural place of power filled with kupuri, just waiting for human beings to embrace it as a way to deal with natural stress. When we have kupuri it replaces stress of all types.

The Health Consequences of Stress

Here is a quick physiology lesson to help give insight into why stress can inhibit your ability to attain optimum health and life balance. Coded into our DNA since ancient times are ways for dealing with just about every stress the natural world can throw at us. Then, as today, responding to challenges was possible because of a hormone called cortisol. Stress of any kind (the result of anything from a charging lion to an irate boss) stimulates the release of this very potent hormone, enabling us to run faster, stay warmer, and have a sharper mind for quick, strategic thinking. Once the stress is over, the levels of cortisol in the blood go back down, and a second hormone called DHEA (dehydroepiandrosterone) is released to bring about a peaceful feeling in your soul. DHEA tells your brain and your heart that everything is okay, that the crisis has passed. DHEA is also responsible for promoting good sleep, building and repairing tissue (including your skin), and keeping your immune system strong and in good working order. It lowers total cholesterol and LDL (the "bad" cholesterol), which helps reduce a person's risk of heart attack.

Unfortunately, in the modern world we deal with challenges nonstop, which means that cortisol is always present and DHEA is often not. Now the trouble begins. When cortisol is continuously around, our bodies are forever in high-alert mode and never in the soothing, hopeful recovery state that we all crave. Since DHEA production is shut down, we no longer have the "life is good" hormone available to signal to every cell in the body that things are okay.

The physical health consequences of a chronically high cortisol level are many:

- Insulin levels rise, which shuts down fat burning.
- Fat is stored around the stomach and in the face.
- New muscle production is stifled.
- Bones become brittle.
- Sleep gets disrupted.
- General energy levels drop.

Long-term stress can also have a heavy impact on emotional health:

- The risk for depression increases.
- Self-esteem lowers.
- Motivation wanes.

- Life seems overwhelming.
- Memory deteriorates.
- Ability to cope with everyday stresses is inhibited.
- Pleasure becomes difficult to experience.

The cumulative effect of all of these symptoms can make you feel lost and sad, and place you in a constant state of worry. The bottom line is that when there is stress, your body tries to respond. At first it will be able to counter the stress without throwing you off balance. But as time goes on, the imbalance that gets set in motion can become increasingly difficult to overcome, making it almost impossible to find happiness and a sense of well-being. This is not because you lack the willpower to push through feelings of fatigue or a lack of motivation—and certainly not because you are weak—but because the elements in your body that give you energy and positive feelings are suppressed.

But take heart. There are simple ways to help identify the sources of stress and bring your body and soul back to the more relaxed state where DHEA is the dominant hormone influencing moods and energy levels. The focus will then be to alleviate the stress, to try to prevent the release of cortisol, and to increase your levels of energy and good feeling with DHEA release. And just as the negatives of stress become cumulative over time, so will the positives of reducing it. Your drive to live life to its fullest will be present more and more, which in turn will fuel a sense of contentment, which gives you more energy and motivation to lead an active life and take care of your soul.

KEY #1:

Balance Your Responses to the Six Types of Stress

The Huichols don't know about cortisol or DHEA, but they are certainly aware of the importance of always working with tools that can reduce stress naturally. One barometer that reveals the Huichols' ability to successfully manage stress is the memory of their elders.

They are rarely affected by Alzheimer's disease in the way that so much of the elderly population in the Western world is. They are able to recall stories and details throughout their entire lives. The shamans, for example, sing thousands of chanted verses that retell their cosmology of creation.

Let's look at the six main types of stress we experience, and then see what can be done to counter them. The lines between these six can get blurred, but there are ways you can target each one individually and bring joy to your body and soul even when you are in the middle of the most difficult workout or an extremely trying period in your life. It's possible to keep focused on your goals for a fit body and soul regardless of the pressures in your life. No situation is hopeless. No one should give up. Every person has a slightly different life situation to work with and challenges that may have to be reversed. You may face barriers that feel impenetrable. They are not.

We'll start with the most prevalent type, emotional stress, and will discuss the step-by-step technique for quieting the mind.

Emotional Stress

Emotional stress is usually what people think of when the word "stress" is mentioned. Very few of us are immune from experiencing it. In fact, one survey found that three-quarters of all adults in America experience great emotional stress weekly. In addition, the other five areas of stress we will talk about all add to one's emotional stress, both because of the hormonal imbalances that get set up through raised cortisol and depressed DHEA, and because of the worry that comes with knowing something is not right in one's body. The longer you feel emotional stress, the more the hormones are released that make it difficult to deal with those stresses. All of the body's coping hormones get depressed, and the pleasure hormones don't get released. This feeds negatively on itself, causing mildly difficult situations to appear insurmountable. Life can seem like a stress-filled nightmare instead of a paradise of wondrous proportions. A fit soul and body this is not.

On the physical level, emotional stress constricts blood vessels, leading to difficulty getting oxygen to working muscles. This also curbs fat metabolism, which is certainly not good for weight control. Emotional stress inhibits the release of human growth hormone, which is required to recover and rebuild your body at the end of each day. It can also lead to feeling burned out, which does not support the motivation we need to exercise daily.

One of the cures for emotional stress is exercise. However, it will be a step forward during the workout, but may be a step backward if the cause of the stress is not improved. This can wind up putting unrealistic pressure on exercise to be the answer to emotional stress, which can lead to added stress when your evening walk or run does not get rid of deadlines, poor working conditions, or a bad family environment. Exercise goals, if unrealistic (wanting results too fast, expecting results that are not within a person's genetic capabilities), can join forces with non-exercise pressures, making it difficult to put a dent in mounting expectations.

Solution: Evict Emotional Stress Using Four Techniques

The solutions to emotional stress are many. The most immediate is to remove the cause of the stress. However, this is often not an option. This brings us to the second solution: alter how we approach, deal with, and are affected by the situations that will be a part of our life. There are four tools we will share with you that will help you respond better to the sources of emotional stress that cannot be eliminated. They are:

- Respond with calmness.
- Clear your mind with laughter.
- Find clarity through the image of the deer.
- Quiet the mind.

Each of these is an ancient tool that effects a positive emotional state by working directly with the needs of a person's soul when it is calling out for help. If we were to watch how a Huichol deals with what could become a very stressful situation, we would see one of these four tools being used to help them diffuse the situation's potentially negative effects.

Respond with Calmness. Job stress is one of the most common ongoing sources of stress for people. Reasons include deadlines, production expectations, employment uncertainty, industry restrictions, and changing work environments. Outside of the work environment people often continue to have to deal with ongoing situations that cause stress, including over-programmed family responsibilities, lack of exercise, and obligations that cut into relaxation time and regenerating activities for your soul.

Fortunately, there are ways to manage these responsibilities and stresses to minimize their negative effect on your life. Deadlines, for example, are a great source of looming stress for nearly everyone— whether you are striving to be in shape for a race, lose a few pounds before an important social event, or finish a project for work. Even the Huichols have deadlines, such as planting when the rains come and harvesting when it's time to gather the crops. Our society is also filled with schedules and timelines that restrict our time and contribute to stress when we let them overwhelm us.

One of the most powerful ways to help shift your response to these challenges is to respond to the stressful situation with calmness. The Huichols understand that they will be under quite a bit of pressure during the planting season each year, as they need to get everything done before the rains come. They acknowledge that each year this stress will exist, and cope with it by approaching every aspect of it with calmness, clearing the land, planting one kernel of corn at a time, until an entire hillside has been sown.

This model of responding with calmness works wonders in the modern world as well. Going back to our example of deadlines, this can help alleviate the stress by acknowledging that, first and foremost, a seemingly overwhelming task does not become finished in one instant. The Huichols don't throw a bushel of corn kernels at the hillside in a panic, in hopes that it will all be planted—quite the opposite. Big projects, from work to fitness gains to changing old patterns about ourselves, all happen one kernel at a time, one step at a time. As each seed is sown, we are one step closer to achieving the goal. Deadline stress most often happens when we search for an unrealistic solution that tries to sidestep this reality. However, if we focus instead on getting the job done in the best way that is possible—one kernel at a time—there is no room for stress. Let calmness reign.

Not everybody has the same strengths or endurance for certain tasks, such as running and walking. But by just doing the best job that you can on any given day with calmness and hope, it shifts your attention, your focus, and your energy away from the stress of performing well, and revives your desire to take the positive action needed to accomplish it. One way to make this shift in focus is to do whatever exercise you are undertaking with the goal of focusing on the mechanics of your movement. If running, be aware of your cadence rate, stride length, and carriage of your shoulders and arms, always striving to find the blend of gait and rhythm that allows your body to feel smooth and at ease. This shifts your focus away from thinking about when the workout will end, from any physical discomfort caused by your level of effort.

A Fit Soul can also provide us with ways to achieve a similar result of feeling at ease rather than pressured to perform, or complete this same task of going for a run. One tool that will be explained in more detail later is learning to focus your attention on the outer environment, especially when you are in naturally beautiful locations. Become aware of the sunlight, its quality on that day. Feel the air around you and the earth beneath your feet. As you run, walk, or sit on the earth, give thanks to the land, mountain, lake, open field, or body of water that you see in your vision. As you become aware of these wonders in nature, your focus shifts away from the stress of performance or finishing anything. The pressures of your life dissipate, and you are infused with good feelings instead.

Clear Your Mind with Laughter. Laughter is an important part of Huichol life and tradition. They say it's a key element to healing, living, and being a whole person. No situation is beyond the bounds of humor for the Huichols. They love to laugh and tease each other and joke around. They see laughter as good medicine: medicine for the soul, and medicine for the body. It's such a simple tool to help shift us toward having positive thoughts and a positive outlook on life. It makes us feel better. For example, as we know when you visit someone in the hospital, if you can bring lightheartedness and humor, even someone who is very sick can feel better on both an emotional and physical level.

Brant's first experience with Huichol humor: When I was first in the Huichol Sierra, a group of us were going to walk to town. It was going to take us about a day to get there. For some reason I was carrying my backpack, which was this huge thing that I had filled to the brim with tons of what certainly had to be useless stuff. It must have weight close to eighty pounds. Coming from America, not only was I not used to carrying heavy loads, I was also unaccustomed to walking such long distances. A day's hike for the Huichols was nothing, but for me it was monumental.

Early in the day we stopped briefly at a beautiful spot to take a break. I was already exhausted. We had most of the day ahead of us, but my big heavy pack and I were ready to call it quits. I had no idea how I was going to make it to our final destination. Sweating and somewhat dejected, I threw the pack down. I was sitting there huffing and puffing, completely absorbed in my situation, when suddenly a Huichol woman in her sixties came over and said, "Oh, do you need help? You look tired!" Without waiting for my response, she grabbed my gigantic pack, slung it onto her back, and ran off. Now my adrenaline was pumping, mostly because I wasn't sure I could keep up with her—even though she was the one with the backpack—but also because I knew this was certainly going to be a scene replayed as something of a comedy skit many, many times around the fire later.

I jumped up and chased after her. I walked behind her for a little while, feeling embarrassed that a sixty-year-old woman was stronger than I was in my twenties. I finally took my backpack back from her. Even to this day, every time I pass by that particular spot on the trail, someone will tease me and ask, "Do you need some help carrying anything?"

When I first brought Don José up to America, there were many cultural differences that stood out for him. One that he commented on right away was that there were very few people just walking around. He asked me, "Where are all the people? Don't they walk?" Don José came from a way of life where people needed to walk as a way to get from one pace to another. But to him, walking was also revered as a simple way to enjoy life. Don José was baffled that people wouldn't want to walk and be outside, even if they did have cars.

On a trip during his later years, he wanted to announce that he was leaving me in his place to carry on the tradition of Huichol shamanism. We visited many places in the U.S.A. and Europe, including different universities. Just before returning to Mexico, we stopped at a bank in San Francisco to change some American money into pesos.

Don José was not fond of huge buildings. So, rather than bring him in with me, we decided he would wait for me outside in the car. I pulled right up in front of the bank and parked. I said, "Don't open the door under any circumstances, no matter what, no matter who

Mark's Use of Laughter

To our sometimes cynical modern ears, this might sound too simplistic—to just laugh your problems away. But for me, laughter helped counter the unrealistic need to have everything go perfectly in my training. Brant healed all of the different physical injuries that I sustained over the course of my triathlon career, and without his power as a healer, I would have missed the final three Ironman Championships that I competed in. But of equal importance in helping me become a champion was the healing of my soul that came from the laughing and teasing that Brant brings as a way of life. It helped get me past the rough patches in my training when things were not going smoothly. I certainly wanted everything to be absolutely perfect, but of course it wasn't. His laughter helped put those moments in perspective.

This lightheartedness has become a requirement between my training partners and me. If one of us was feeling good, we would laugh about that. If one of us was feeling good and another not so good, we would laugh even more. If we all felt lousy, that would get us rolling on the ground in hysterics. Of course we always want to feel a thousand percent when we're training, but that just isn't the reality. And we needed to shift our focus away from something that certainly could have been perceived as stressful and place it on something joyous—like laughter.

comes by. It's a wild city here in San Francisco." I was nervous because I had this great, great shaman and Huichol chief, a very revered shaman and elder, in my care. He was my responsibility. I left him in the car and went into the bank.

Fortunately, when I came back out he was still sitting there in the car and everything looked just like it had when I left him. I opened the door so he could get out. We wanted to take a little walk. As I opened the door for him, he said, "Hey, some nice policeman came by. He was smiling at me and I smiled back at him. But I think he might have known you, maybe he was your friend. He came by three times, and each time he wrote you a letter and left it under the windshield wiper. One glance at the front of the car revealed the nice "letters" I had been left . . . three tickets!

I always remember this story because it showed the innocence of the Huichols, and especially of Don José. He had never gotten a ticket in his life, never driven a car himself. Humor is such an important part of their daily life and even at their sacred ceremonies. We always joke around. A lot of their ceremonial deer dances last all night, accompanied by sacred songs and folk songs. Then during the breaks we tell stories and jokes and laugh a lot. Stress is simply not present.

Have you ever noticed that when a person is happy and laughing he or she seems to shine with a brightness of spirit? This is nature's beauty treatment for body and soul. Laughter dissipates stress and frees the mind. The Huichols use laughter over and over again each day of their lives as a way to rid themselves of fear and depression, and to shift their focus away from what causes them stress and replace it with hope. Even in modern societies, laughter has been acknowledged as a healing medicine. You know yourself that if you're visiting someone who is unhappy and you can make them laugh, they feel better. This is another simple, powerful, natural tool you can use to dispel emotional stress.

Find Clarity Through the Image of the Deer. Another way to dissipate emotional stress is to connect with the part of your being that houses love—your heart. The Huichols use the image of the deer to represent gentleness, innocence, and clarity. We believe the deer is part of our higher self, the part of us that knows everything already and is inherently connected not only intuitively to every cell in our body, but also ultimately connected to the universe and all of creation. The deer can bring you balance, healing, and well-being. The deer is a higher power of one's self. This strong but gentle deer spirit is your center and can give you answers to problems that can be causing you emotional stress.

Invoking the Image of the Deer

To begin this exercise, find a comfortable place to stand or sit. Bring the image of a deer surrounded by a circle into your consciousness. You may also try to find a sense of peace as you do this exercise, as peace or harmony with your world or environment is your ultimate goal. It might be seen as similar to meditation (an image of peace). You will be asking the deer for guidance when your mind cannot solve life's mysteries. A Huichol would use the deer to help him or her through tough times in his or her life.

Call out, "Hey deer spirit person, deer essence, my higher self, help me! Help me to hold on to my vision of balance and harmony. Help me to hold onto my vision of Fit Soul, Fit Body. Don't let me fall. Help me to stand up tall like a tree reaching up to the sky." You may say this out loud or meditate silently with these thoughts. Even the Huichols are sometimes self-conscious, and may prefer to do things silently.

Let yourself be a bridge between the worlds of earth and sky, between your inner world and the outer environment. Focus on this as your reality and remember that your life is something sacred. You are part of something wondrous.

Allow the stress to leave and to have beauty, power, and joy come into your heart. Imagine a beautiful image of nature coming and nurturing your body. Feel the power of this transformation and ultimately the joy that materializes as a result of your sincere efforts.

KEY #2:

Quiet the Mind

This technique is so powerful that we're calling it a main key; it's helpful even when stress is not a factor. Your thoughts become your reality, both in the positive and negative sense. For example, think of two people jogging the same distance together. One might feel like he went a little farther than he had expected to on that day and be elated with the surprise addition to his workout. The second might feel like the run was a little shorter than she had hoped it to be and feel disappointed and stressed because she didn't do enough. Which one do you think will absorb that workout the best and be excited and motivated from it? Who will experience stress from it?

Certainly not every day will bring pleasant surprises, like an easier time at work or a more fulfilling walk or run than expected. So when life seems to be falling short, our fourth tool to help you deal with emotional stress is learning to quiet your mind. This is an extremely effective tool for dissipating emotional stress and helping to shift negative thoughts. When your mind is quiet, you stop viewing a situation as stressful. The place to find this quiet is in calmness of spirit. In modern terminology this means stopping the dialogue inside your head. Normally we are always rearranging things with our thoughts. We have conversations with people where we might not like what transpired, and later in our mind we mull over old situations, changing what they said, then what we said. Look at all the energy that is consumed in order for us to keep our minds working! When this energy is focused on negative situations, it is exhausting and stressful.

Silencing the Mind Exercise

For many of us, the only alteration we can make to the stresses in our lives is to change how we view them. Often our reaction to a situation is what makes it good or bad. We may not be able to find a new boss, work less, or stop dealing with deadlines. But we can simply exercise as a way to reduce stress. When anticipating a workout or race, just like any situation that causes stress, remember what your original reasons were that sparked you to exercise. Use those as a way to shift your response. This will help DHEA, the feel-good hormone, keep flowing, and will curb the release of cortisol, the on-alert hormone.

The Huichols practice this model every day, often going out to gather firewood or water as a way to get some exercise and take a break from what might be causing them stress. They also strive to focus on positive feelings.

This exercise, which is akin to meditation, soothes your soul and can help shift how you respond to a potentially stressful situation, simply by quieting the part of your mind that would indeed say "This is stressful."

When you need to quiet negative thoughts that are running through your mind, follow these steps:

1. Start by sitting down in a comfortable spot outside. If you can, find a special place that nourishes your whole being, preferably a quiet place surrounded by nature. If this is not possible, find a place with grass or a tree, or any place that feels good to you. If you don't know of one yet, discover a place for yourself that nurtures each part of who you are: your body, your heart, your spirit, and your soul. Let yourself be drawn to a beautiful area in nature.

2. Visualize a sacred circle that connects you to all of life in front of your heart. This is called the *nerika* (see nerika exercise on page 68). The nerika is a doorway, a visionary link to all of creation. It can be seen as coming from your heart and is also akin to a mirror reflecting knowledge or feelings from us to everyone and everything. The nerika is in the mystical air we all breathe and can also be felt as awareness. Remember, the heart is connected to the mind and can actually be thought of as one and the same. Visualize yourself going into that circle of light and energy coming from your heart.

3. Next, stop the stream of thoughts in your mind. Go to a place between the worlds of distraction and imbalance, or an internal place between the thoughts that might interfere with feeling balance, to a place of silence. Between two thoughts there is a certain silence, a certain peace. Let the tranquility that emerges from this place of silence fill your spirit.

4. Try to avoid developing new thoughts. When a thought tries to come into your consciousness, gently deflect it. You have already visualized yourself inside the nerika; continue to imagine your heat and your being inside of the circle, the circle of life. Stay in its center. Visualize yourself surrounded by light and color, and empower your soul. Look for a certain silence; feel the peace that is inside. Don't think about it. Just feel it.

You don't necessarily have to be sitting in a comfortable spot to do this exercise successfully. It comes in handy during all kinds of scenarios, and you can practice it during stressful situations, just as Mark did during his Ironman races. The key is to replace stressful or negative thoughts with positive, peaceful ones and use the beauty in your surroundings—or even what you can create in your mind—to bring this about.

Sleep Deprivation Induced Stress

Sleep, nourishing sleep! The spirit of regeneration works upon each and every person during sleep. Every cell in your body, every part of you, gets regenerated during this time. The Huichols say that when sleeping, you die a little death—you go to the Great Spirit, or to a special place of power, where everything just *is*. Without this deep, uninterrupted form of sleep, you cannot regenerate your body and soul to the fullest.

Without adequate amounts of restorative sleep, our bodies release cortisol, which sets up a stress cycle and causes a disruption in the sleep we do get. Elevated cortisol also leads to a slowing-down of your body's fat-burning capabilities. So if you are trying to lose those final pounds and cannot, try looking at your sleep patterns. If you are not getting enough, add in some extra hours or minutes every night to help you reach your goal.

Sleep is natural medicine, pure and simple! Without enough quality sleep, you cannot regenerate physically or emotionally. You won't produce human growth hormone, which is needed to regenerate muscle tissue. A lot of aging is a function of a lifetime of continual, low-grade stress that eventually robs the brain of sleep and memory and the body of the time it needs to regenerate. A person with disrupted sleep and the resulting low DHEA levels will start to become forgetful and confused. This makes it even more difficult to figure out what needs to be done to improve fitness and health.

Perhaps the most significant effect of sleep deprivation is the disruption of your energy cycles. If you aren't getting enough sleep, you may find that you are tired in the middle of the day, but wired late at night. You may go to sleep easily but wake up much earlier than expected and not be able to get back to sleep. Or you may get what seems to be a normal amount of sleep but then wake up tired, not feeling refreshed.

Being physically and mentally fatigued makes it difficult to take the time to make the positive connections with life that feed your soul and heal your body. You can then feel completely overwhelmed just trying to deal with life. You might feel burdened by responsibilities rather than happy to take the time to share joy with others in both your workouts and your life.

Solution: Prepare for a Good Night's Sleep

Here are a few sleepy-time tips to help make your slumber deep and regenerative:

- Keep caffeine consumption limited to the early parts of the day (before noon).
- Avoid big meals late in the day, which can set up blood sugar swings and wake you up in the night when insulin is overdoing its job. Adopt a simple practice the Huichols use, which is to eat a light dinner many days of the week.
- Keep alcohol consumption, if any, in the healthy zone (around one drink a night). Excessive alcohol causes a hormone to be released in the middle of the night that actually wakes you up, causing disrupted sleep.
- Try to leave worries from the day behind so your mind is free when you hit the pillow. Sleep time is for *sleep*, not for figuring out how you will deal with life's challenges. Go over the day's events and then just let them go into an imaginary sacred circle in front of your heart. This helps you prepare to go into deep sleep without being held back by the day's events.

Dietary Stress

We'll be going into optimum diet choices in Chapter 6, but here's a brief introduction to food's power on our bodies and souls as it relates to stress.

Food is nourishing and necessary to our bodies. However, an unbalanced diet causes stress in the body: Eating too little or too much of even the healthiest foods will cause a cascade of negatives that can disrupt your digestive system and hinder your body's ability to recover from exercise or just a long day at work. It can also cause emotional instabilities that make it tough to maintain a positive outlook on life. Take protein, for example. By eating less than your body needs for daily recovery and repair, you can feel hungry no matter how many other calories you eat, simply because your body is searching for a major nutrient that is missing. But consume too much protein and the kidneys are under a huge stress, excreting nitrogen byproducts of dietary protein.

If you eat too few good fats and oils, you won't be able to make the hormones that keep your body working properly, your skin will be less healthy, and sexual function can be disrupted. Too many fats, especially the saturated ones, and not only will excess weight become an issue, but the unseen deterioration of the cardiovascular system can be set in motion. Too few carbohydrates or too many carbohydrates in your diet both lead to a state where you constantly crave carbs. A significant lack of overall calories (more than 10–15 percent less than your daily caloric requirement) and your body goes into lack-of-calorie stress, which slows down the metabolic engine in your body, causing weight gain, lowered energy levels, difficulty concentrating, and mood swings. Too many calories or only eating one or two meals each day (even if the number of calories is enough), and weight gain also becomes likely, as well as highs and lows in energy, focus, and mood.

Solution: Let Dietary Habits Be an Antidote to—Not a Stimulator of—Stress

Following are some dietary tips that will help limit the amount of stress the foods you eat cause your body. For a complete discussion of the right kind of diet to help you achieve a Fit Soul and Fit Body, see Chapter 6.

- Avoid simple sugars and choose carbohydrates that are from whole grains, fresh vegetables, and small amounts of fruit. If you choose to indulge in simple sugars on occasion, make sure you don't eat the sugar on an empty stomach: have a little bit of protein, healthy oils, and complex carbs in your system already, so the sugar won't cause a dramatic increase in insulin levels. This will help you to regulate your mood and accompanying motivation.
- Cut back on or cut out caffeine. In moderate amounts, such as two cups of coffee a day, caffeine is fine in an unstressed person. But in an overstressed body, it will destabilize blood sugar even more.
- Add some healthy oils—like cold pressed olive oil or omega-3 oil—to your meals to help balance your hormones.
- Ensure you are getting the right amount of protein in your diet (a full discussion of your personal dietary needs will follow in Chapter 6). This not only helps build new muscle, but also counters the effects of too many carbohydrates.
- Eat a good breakfast within an hour of so of waking, and eat frequent small meals throughout the day (at least every three to four hours).

Physical Stress

This kind of stress typically occurs from exerting yourself too much in a workout, but it also affects those who have the type of job that demands a lot physically, such as a construction workers, manual laborers, or plant employees. What this kind of stress means will be different for each person, depending on your overall health and life stress. If we lived in a tent on a mountain and had no responsibilities other than using our bodies physically, the volume and intensity of exercise that we could endure would be tremendous. However, in the real world of jobs, family, and other stresses, physically over-working or overtraining can cause sickness, injury, or burnout. Here are some distinct signs that indicate the amount of physical work you are doing is beyond your body's ability to absorb the benefits. If you are experiencing any of them, it's time for a reality check: You are most likely suffering from physical stress.

- A waking heart rate that is elevated more than five beats above normal. (While it may not be practical to test your heart rate every morning, if you sense that your heart is beating at an elevated clip when you wake up, it may be time to check it, using a heart rate monitor kept by your bedside.)
- General irritability.
- Inability to sleep soundly even after strenuous exercise or physical labor.
- Loss of appetite, especially compared to what you normally need for your exercise level.
- Overall fatigue that lasts more than two or three days.
- Chronic muscle soreness.
- Lack of motivation to train or do anything physical lasting more than two or three days.
- Injury.
- Illness.

We will give you guidelines for conditioning your body that will help you make exercise a stress reducer rather than a stress enhancer in Chapter 5. This will be important for sustaining your journey to a Fit Body as well as a Fit Soul. If ignored, any one of the signs of physical stress can lead to emotional states that are the opposite of the goal of having a Fit Soul. Some of these are:

- Depression.
- Inability to concentrate.
- Low self-esteem.
- Self-doubt.
- Unprovoked fear.
- Feeling too paralyzed to take action.

As you can see, each of these should be relieved through exercise. Yet, overdoing it physically could bring them out rather than eliminate them.

Solution: Be Mindful of the Signs of Physical Stress

These tips will help you monitor the intensity of your workout and ensure that you are not overtraining.

- If you feel that your exercise routine may be too intense for you, use a heart rate monitor while exercising so that you can keep your heart in a healthy and mostly fat-burning zone (see Chapter 5).
- Gauge your level of day-to-day fatigue from exercise as well as your overall recovery rate by checking for the signs of overexertion listed above. It may help to keep a journal and track your daily energy levels. If any of the symptoms above start to describe you, it's time to cut back on the overall volume and training intensity, and get some rest until the signs are no longer there.

Always remember to assess your current state based on how you really feel, rather than how you *think* you should feel. Each day, week, and year in a person's life is different, and it's impossible to assume that what might have been a manageable amount of exercise at another time in your life will still work today.

As an aside, bear in mind that your body may sense physical stress from the rigors of your daily life regardless of your exercise regimen. In other words, if you can check off the symptoms listed above and don't engage in physical exercise much, clearly this is a sign that your life could be out of balance. In these cases, you would do well to incorporate *more* exercise into your schedule and pinpoint areas in your life that are dragging you down, depleting your energy, and preventing you from finding that perfect balance whereby physical stress is minimized and health and wellness are maximized.

Chemical Stress

Chemical stress occurs when your body has to get rid of compounds that are harmful or toxic to it. Most toxins that create chemical stress come from the external environment—everything from the air you breathe to the water and food you eat to the home you live in can be a source of harmful chemicals.

Here are three of the most commonplace things that can cause chemical stress:

1. **Caffeine.** In small doses (two cups of coffee or less per day) caffeine can actually stimulate fat burning and heighten mental acuity. However, in excess, this potent chemical—which works by stimulating the adrenal system—can cause long-term exhaustion, emotional edginess, disrupted or restless sleep, and destabilized blood sugar levels, which causes cravings for the goodies that neither rebuild the body or help with weight loss.

2. **Alcohol.** Again, if the alcohol is consumed in small quantities (up to two drinks for men and one for women daily), most people will be fine. Alcohol can increase HDL (high- density lipoprotein, the good form of cholesterol in your blood) and block the formation of LDL (low-density lipoprotein, the bad form of cholesterol in your blood). This, coupled with red wine's antioxidant properties, can reduce your risk of a heart attack by 30–50 percent. However, this is not an endorsement to go out and grab a glass of wine. Alcohol consumption is also associated with increased triglycerides and fat gain around the midsection, neither of which is a plus for health, exercising, or feeling good. And as far as the antioxidant properties, blueberries stand head and shoulders above red wine in this category.

3. **Sugar.** In small quantities, and when eaten with other foods, sugar's ill effects are reduced. However, "sugar" and "small quantities" rarely go together. This chemical (yes, it is a chemical) is infamous for causing weight gain, food cravings, and mood swings, and for reducing the desire for the foods that help build a healthy, active body, such as protein and good oils (omega-3 especially). We will cover this topic in depth in Chapter 6.

Solution: Reduce Your Exposure to Toxins

Food can be one of the main methods through which environmental chemicals enter your body, and is also the one that you have the most control over. Eating foods without insecticides or chemical additives and drinking pure water are two good ways to start reducing the amount of harmful toxins your body will have to filter out. This means seeking out foods that are grown organically and that are free of artificial compounds. Read the ingredient lists on the packaging of your food. Labels that list items you could actually purchase yourself are probably healthy. The more exotic or difficult to pronounce an ingredient is, the higher the chance that it is a chemical your body will not be fond of. By choosing good foods, your body can use its energy to take in nutrients instead of having to get rid of what is artificial.

Environmental toxins (things like poor air quality and building materials) may not show their negative effects in your body for some time. Some of the negative effects include: feeling weak when you enter a room or office; sudden stuffiness, running nose, or watering eyes and itchy skin. You may have much less control over your exposure to these chemicals than you do over the food you eat, but, as always, the cleaner your immediate environment, the easier it will be for your body to do the job it is supposed to. Cleaning up the air you breathe and the water you drink is as easy as investigating good water-filtration systems, choosing all-natural cleaning supplies, letting your home aerate by opening up the windows during the day, and being mindful of what you put on your skin in the form of body-care products and cosmetics, which may contain a host of toxic chemicals. We live at a time when there are a growing number of alternatives to chemical-based products. You don't have to live in a bubble to reduce your risk of exposure to noxious chemicals. You simply have to be a conscientious consumer and opt for organic, all-natural products whenever possible.

Inflammation Induced Stress

Inflammation has become a buzzword in medical circles, but people don't normally think of inflammation as a cause of stress to the body.

They see it only as an effect of stress, when in fact it's a little of both—a signal *and* promoter of stress on the body. So too much inflammation can be a vicious cycle. As the inflammation responds to stress, it also creates more stress if left unchecked.

There is such a thing as good inflammation—the kind you get if you cut your hand, for example, when redness and swelling soon follows. This kind of inflammation helps prevent further injury to the site and causes the immune system to come take action to hasten the healing process. The inflammatory response is the body's first line of defense against injury and infection, and that pain and heat you feel after an injury is a sign that your body is working. But an out-of-control inflammatory response can destroy healthy tissue and cause more damage than the original problem. Keeping it under control means the immune system must maintain a balance between fanning the flames of inflammation and cooling it down.

Signs of so-called bad inflammation include sore or stiff joints (something that many people consider a normal part of aging, but that is often a simple sign of excess inflammation)—which certainly don't fuel the desire to exercise. Inflammation also affects the brain by restricting blood vessels, reducing blood flow, and often causing headaches, which again reduces our sense of feeling good and being motivated to approach life. Detectable conditions such as cancer, arthritis, heart disease, Alzheimer's, allergies, and many autoimmune diseases are all links to internal inflammation, which causes cortisol to be released. And as you have learned, this can lead to low motivation, malaise, and fatigue of the body and soul.

Inflammation can come from a number of things, including minor infections, too many overly intense workouts, being overweight, or eating foods that upset the digestive tract. Inflammation can become chronic if a person eats too much saturated fat and not enough omega-3 (cold-water fish and flaxseed oil). Even normally healthy oils like canola oil will be converted to a form that causes inflammation if a person is under stress.

Solution: Tame the Flames of Bad Inflammation

Inflammation is initially less noticeable than sickness, injury, or burnout (physical stress) or feelings of being overwhelmed, depressed, or unmotivated (emotional stress). A stiff joint is usually not a big red flag for people that there needs to be lifestyle changes. Alzheimer's is a big red flag, but once the disease has set in it is usually too late to reverse, even if the inflammation is reduced. So here are a few preventative measures that will help keep you away from inflammation stress:

- Balance your fat intake. Reduce saturated fats and oils containing omega-6 (canola or soy oil), and increase your dietary amount of omega-3 oils (fish oil, flaxseed oil, walnuts, beans) and olive oil. See Chapter 6 for more details about optimum diet choices.
- Continue with consistent, moderate heart-rate exercise to help reduce overall weight if this is an issue.
- Limit yourself to a moderate intake of carbohydrates. Moderating carbohydrates in your diet can help promote fat burning in your body, which in turn reduces inflammation. Aerobic exercise reduces the level of insulin, a hormone that constricts all your blood vessels. When your blood vessels open up, inflammation is naturally reduced. (Much more to come on choosing optimum foods and healthy carbohydrates in Chapter 6.)
- Omit foods from your diet that cause discomfort or digestive problems. If you feel tired or weak, get the sniffles, become bloated after eating, or have severe negative reactions to particular foods, chances are they are not healthy foods for you. Most common among these are shellfish, meat, eggs, dairy, soy, wheat, some fruits, and nuts.

Exercise: A Common Denominator in Stress Reduction

The stress-relieving exercises in this book will help you calm your mind and relax so that you can concentrate your energy on the important things in your life, including your fitness program. Remember that a balanced workout program can be your ally in your battle against all types of stress. Moderate exercise, like walking, can be the key to overcoming the negativity and fatigue that so often accompany stress. The Huichols use walking as a natural way to relieve stress and as a special chance to gain kupuri (life force) by simply feeling their connection to the earth and to nature as they walk.

Sometimes you can find yourself paralyzed by the feeling of being too tired to work out, yet too wired to get the sleep you need to regenerate your body. Studies have shown a direct correlation between quality of sleep and working out, but what can you do when you find yourself with this conundrum?

Even if you feel you are too tired to do anything physical, one of the best ways to try to regain your energy is to engage in a moderate workout, even if it's just for a short amount of time. Set aside about twenty minutes to move your body at a very easy pace. Stay away from trying to hit the high end of your workout heart rates right now. The relaxed nature of this workout will reduce stress hormones in your system and stimulate the release of the ones that make you happy and peaceful. Continue the light workout for at least three consecutive days and take note of its effect on your sleep patterns. Just a little exercise can go a long way toward bringing back peaceful sleep.

Moderate aerobic exercise lowers levels of cortisol and elevates DHEA, the happiness and anti-aging hormone. Working out won't take away the external stresses, like a big credit card bill, but it will help counteract the stress response in your body. By exercising, you set in motion the rebalancing of your internal environment so that instead of seeing the world as a stressful place to exist, you can be overwhelmed with the beauty that surrounds you every moment of the day.

Remember, too, that the Fit Soul exercises for reducing stress can work in tandem with your workouts. You can, for example, plan a hike or nature walk with a close friend. Not only will you be engaged physically, but you can also use the time to quiet your mind, enjoy a few laughs, and find refuge from the stress of daily life just by being present together and surrounded by the beauty of nature. In the next chapter you'll learn additional Fit Soul techniques that will enhance the quality of your life and activities while helping you to further conquer overall stress. Transforming negative emotions into positive ones using tried and true strategies to complement your stress-reduction techniques.

A realistic and active approach to stress will open the gates to a world where you can achieve what you want, shape up your body and spirit, and cultivate an attitude that brings you good feelings about life—no matter what happens. Some stresses may never go away, but hopefully by being active in your use of the tools that alleviate their effects, they won't hold you back from good health and peace of mind. Stress, up to a point, is actually good for a human being. A healthy dose of physical stress, for instance, is what we call a workout and is what makes you faster, stronger, quicker, and more flexible. A moderate amount of emotional stress keeps us from getting lazy and helps us finish projects, create new ideas, focus intently, and learn. The tools you now have at hand will keep you in the healthy zone that invigorates and motivates you in life.

Chapter Three
Manage Obstacles
to Well-Being

You can be fearless and have still have a little fear. Do not surrender to fear, but go through it with dignity and grace.

One of the most fearsome experiences can be standing at the start of a big race. Picture yourself in a moment like that, even if you've never raced before. You're surrounded by other athletes—all of whom you think are better, faster, and more fit than you. The start line of the Ironman is particularly terrifying. No one is fooling around in this competition. Fifteen hundred fiercely competitive athletes who qualified to get here are salivating for a win. Ahead of us lies 140 miles of swimming, biking, and running in weather conditions that you know will seem insurmountable. Every time I competed in the Ironman, fear would well up inside of me. I felt completely vulnerable to the thought that I had not done enough of the right kind of training to get my body ready. Everyone else seemed more prepared than I was. I trembled at the idea of not knowing where I would possibly find the strength of soul to make it through the thousands of moments when my body would scream out for me to stop.

This fear could have been paralyzing, except for this simple teaching from Brant: "**Be fearless in the face of your fears**." Repeating this spoke a thousand words to my soul and gave me strength. Being fearless in the face of all those fears gave me the confidence and trust I needed to go forward anyway—no matter what. Once I learned this mantra, I began using it in all sorts of situations, many of which had nothing to do with racing or getting ready for the gun to go off.

Another technique that I learned on the racecourse to replace negative chatter with peaceful thoughts has also become a regular practice for me in a variety of situations. This was briefly mentioned in the previous chapter: using the image of the nerika, which you'll learn how to do in greater detail in this chapter. It was particularly important in 1992, when I competed in the biggest triathlon on the European continent—the Nice Triathlon in France. This event takes place in one of the most beautiful places on earth. The swim is in the powder-blue waters of the Mediterranean Sea, the bike winds through the foothills of the Maritime Alps, and the run passes along the beach-lined Côte d'Azur. It sounds idyllic until you find yourself seven minutes behind the French champion with less than ten miles to go in the race.

To make up that much time with so little racing left was nearly impossible, and certainly would have been if I had allowed myself to give up, which wouldn't have been hard to do at that point. But just like any time I wanted to give up, I realized I had forgotten to focus on joy, hope, or gratitude, teachings that Brant emphasized as a simple tool that can pull you out of extremely tough moments. The only way to rediscover that in the heat of an impossible comeback was to go into the nerika, that place of the heart that is naturally calm and alert. I was lucky to have practiced this over and over under Brant's tutelage during retreats and at other times that were peaceful and joyful. Now was the test to see if I could do it under pressure.

So that's what I did. I concentrated my focus on the circle in front of my heart that is a place of silence and calm. The negative thoughts melted away. This quieted my mind and helped me to feel happy just to be in the race. Bit by bit, I closed in on my opponent. Being a Frenchman racing in his hometown, he was surrounded by thousands of fans cheering him to what appeared to be certain victory. But with less than four hundred meters to go, I passed him, still in that place of calm and enthusiasm, and was able to come back from behind to claim the championship. It was one of ten championships I won in this annual race. Luckily, I never lost a single race I started in Nice, thanks in large part to a Fit Soul.

When Negative Emotions Run Deep

Creating a new model of health and wellness for our lives is much the same as the process of remodeling a home that no longer serves our needs. First we look at what part of the structure will have to be taken down and cleared away so that a new, better, sturdier, more functional, and beautiful space can take form. If we're lucky, the things needed to complete this task are cosmetic, like a new coat of paint. Other times we need to disassemble everything, all the way down to the foundation, if we are going to build a lasting structure for the vision we have.

Our bodies and souls are the same. If the old model of living is not getting you to the level you want, it might be a call for a completely new paradigm of how to live. If your soul cannot find peace and happiness, and does not feel energy for life, it might be time for a new approach to the world and your connection to it.

We need body and soul to be working together from the ground up. All the lifestyle choices in the world will be placed on a shaky foundation if one's focus in life lacks a positive nature. Likewise, no amount of imagery can heal a sedentary body that is being plagued by poor eating habits and unhealthy decisions. In both cases, the old must be cleared away if it is going to support that wonderful state of being that is healthy, happy, and complete.

The last chapter's discussion of stress gave you tools to help clear away outside influences that can get in the way of this purpose. Now let's look inward and find the keys necessary to rebuild a new body from the inside out—from the soul outward. The most significant of these is going to be developing ways to clear out negative emotions and then replace them with empowering ones.

Are your emotions generally positive? Do you take solace in personal confidence? Is your focus on boredom and doubt or on possibility and positive outcomes? These are just three questions that will be addressed in the upcoming pages.

You have probably experienced how significant your thoughts are at influencing whether or not you feel motivated to give 100 percent. Positive thoughts give you energy, trust, and hope for change, which can cause long periods where life seems easy to navigate. Thinking good thoughts brings peace to your soul and gives you confidence in life. The Huichols understand the importance of having a good attitude, and they work to transform three basic negative emotions that can hold all human beings back. These are:

- Fear
- Anger
- Jealousy

The list of emotions we could look at is a long one, but the Huichols say that all other negative emotions can be traced back to one of these three. If you live your life in fear, it can stifle your ability to take positive action. If you pay attention to anger, you will attract anger and everything will make you irritated. If you become envious of someone else's good fortune, it can rip your heart apart and distract you from your own goals. Learning how to cope with and resolve these negative feelings allows the joy, power, and health of your body and soul to flourish.

KEY #3:

Transform Fear, Anger, and Jealousy

Good thoughts lead us to incredible awareness and experiences. This truth can be learned and experienced by everyone. Athletes know this, and they do everything they can to psych themselves up for big sporting events like the Olympics. They shake their arms and legs. They jump up and down to keep loose and relaxed. They listen to their favorite music or hide under a towel as a way to shut out distractions. They all want to feel "up" when the starting gun goes off. Each day in our own lives is filled with personal Olympic moments when we have a task ahead that we want to do well and know it is going to take being "up" to make it happen. The task is irrelevant; it could be an important meeting, a big workout, a running race, a tough but necessary talk with a friend, or a commitment to a daily spiritual practice. Each of these events will be richer if our emotional state is positive. Fear, anger, or jealousy are not emotions that will help us in these important moments, nor will they help us in simple day-to-day tasks.

Fizzle Out Fear

We all have felt fear when faced with challenges. It is a normal emotion. Fear even has a positive purpose, as it keeps us safe and out of harm's way. But when it holds you back from doing what is important, whether switching careers or facing life with truth, you can profit from changing the response to fear—which might paralyze you from taking action—and shift that feeling of wanting to run and hide so that the desire to go forward in life is strong, even in the face of fear.

Many times the fear that you won't be able to achieve what you want causes a loss of enthusiasm and motivation. One deceptively simple technique the Huichols use to cope with fear is to shift the focus of the mind away from fear and doubt. You can make this shift by focusing on a positive event in the natural world that will continue on whether you face your fear or not. The moment fear starts to creep in, recall the colors of the last sunrise or sunset that gave your soul comfort and strength. Let your attention be directed for a moment to the season you are in and how it will continue on regardless of whether you have fear or lack self-confidence.

Sound simple? It is, but try it. Doing this brings a bigger perspective to a personal outcome that you might be worried about. Winning a race or succeeding in anything you set out to do is fantastic, but fearing failure will not change the fact that the rain will fall and the sun will rise. Let these images remind you that we are all part of something big and grand. Allow this to bring trust into your own life. Let fear take a backseat, so that you can take action even if the fear is still there. This is what we call being fearless in the face of your fear.

Solution: Be Fearless in the Face of Your Fears

This skill, like any, takes practice. Here are a few real-life examples that can help you to master being fearless in the face of your fears, so that you can be propelled forward in your life rather than stifled by it.

- **Bite off a smaller chunk**. Often fear comes when we feel overwhelmed by the task—or series of tasks—ahead. It can be anything from losing lots of weight to re-training yourself in a new professional area, from doing an Ironman to changing old patterns that you have relied on for years. When the job seems too big and fear pops up telling us it's hopeless or impossible, shift the fear by breaking down the task into the smallest steps you can manage, so you can actually see yourself accomplishing them one at a time.

- **Take the first step**. The unknown ferments in the mind when fear is present. We create scenarios filled with obstacles, convinced that each one will bring certain doom. Thinking about what lies ahead can be paralyzing. So take the first step, then the next, and then the one after that. Suddenly you will see that all the things that caused you so much fear are actually far easier to deal with in the real world than in your imagination. (And all those steps add up!)

- **Accept the fact that challenge is normal**. Everyone has self-confidence when everything goes smoothly. Fear can come up when the bumps in the road get big and we just want to slam on the brakes rather than figuring out how to get past them and keep going. Challenge is normal. Realizing this will help you manage obstacles. Seeing challenge as a tool for learning can propel you forward in your search for a healthy soul. As Billie Jean King said, "Pressure is a privilege."

- **Be fearless in the face of your fears**. This is a very powerful teaching that comes from the Huichols. What it means is to keep going with what is important even if you feel fear in the moment. It is a credo that reminds us that even if we have fear, it doesn't have to hold us back. Go to the start line of a race—or a job opportunity, or a chance to meet someone new, whatever—even if you are terrified of it. Start lines don't have to be race-related; they are metaphors for saying yes to fresh and thrilling new experiences. Go into the health club and start those workouts you have feared for months. Have the tough talk that you have avoided with a distanced loved one. Remember that talk the next time fear causes you to hesitate. Be fearless in the face of your fears and take that step anyway. More than likely, the outcome will be something wonderful, something that propels you to a new chapter in life that's better, more satisfying, and definitely more enriching.

Letting Nature Transform Fear

A negative emotion such as fear can affect many different areas of your life. Fearing that you may not get the promotion that you want could hold you back from taking the steps to do so. Fearing you will have a very tough time in a workout or a race can make your body tight enough that it does become a supreme challenge. Fearing that a relationship with a loved one is falling apart may keep you from finding the right words to mend it.

Here is an exercise to help you transform fear into power and courage. It is okay to have fear; however, we can also use fear as a way to empower us. Do not succumb to fear, even if you are afraid. We have all had these feelings at different times in our life.

Seek out a place in nature where you can surround yourself with the beauty of things that are not man-made and feel a connection to all of life. A good place would be a park, under a tree, even on the grass in your backyard. You are a part of all life and should not be afraid of it. Embrace the silence and let it wash away anxieties and fear.

Then, when night falls, go somewhere where the only light comes from the stars overhead. Embrace the darkness. Welcome the darkness and the silence into your life as a natural aspect of our environment. Listen to the silence, to that natural form of darkness. The darkness of nature is also a part of who you are. If you are not able to go to an isolated place in nature, you can also do this exercise near your house in as quiet and dark a place as possible. If you are afraid of the dark and cannot get past that fear, it's okay to try this exercise with dim lighting. Focus less on the darkness and more on the quiet. Listen to the safe sounds of nature around you. ⚘

Employ the Light of the Sun

Another way to work with fear is to go out and honor the rising sun. Bring the light and warmth into your body, into your soul, and into your spirit. Really *feel* that connection by opening your heart and soul and let a feeling of love for the warmth and the light of the sun take over your emotions. Concentrate on the light. The light transforms the darkness of night into the brilliance of day. Witnessing this transformation brings courage to your soul and brightness to your being. ⚘

Evict Anger

Think of the last time you were angry. Was it today, yesterday, or can't you remember because it was so long ago? Most people can pinpoint the last time they were angry; it's a powerful emotion that, for some, surfaces regularly. Anger can rob the vital energy we need for the important steps we want to take toward good health. Don José Matsuwa often said that anger is not who you are. There are lots of things that can make people angry. The one we want to address is the anger that comes when you can't seem to make the changes in either body or soul that you want. It's a feeling that you will never, ever be able to make the physical and emotional changes you have worked so hard for.

One way to shift away from the frustration or anger is to trust in a timeline of change that is real, one that is in sync with the slow change that takes place in nature.

The modern world does not support this concept: On television we see transformations that seem to happen almost instantly and without effort. All the time, we hear things like: "Lose fifty pounds in six weeks, guaranteed!" "Take charge of your life and your finances immediately with this simple new system! Empower yourself instantly." None of these statements has value based in sustainability over time. Our attention span has sunk to such a low level that it exists almost exclusively in a state of impatience. We can't wait for anything. Expecting changes in body and soul instantly can be as frustrating as the slow progress of a traffic jam on the freeway.

Having a Fit Soul and a Fit Body is something to aspire to over an entire lifetime, not just a couple of weeks. This perspective helps in the moments when you might want to throw in the towel because the changes you are making are at a snail's pace. The only requirement for a Fit Soul and a Fit Body is to get back up and keep on going.

Solution: Transforming Anger to Trust

Your journey started with the belief that change is indeed possible. When it seems it is not, here are a few thoughts to bring it back.

- Feeling frustrated because you've been doing the work to change, but nothing seems to be happening? Trust in yourself, in your environment, and in your ability to live a healthier, more empowered life. "I can and I will" says a thousand words to your soul. It renews the possibility of transformation.
- Is your anger telling your hand to grab the food that will work against your body-change goals? Stop, and then trust that over time the weight will come off. Trust that tomorrow you will have the desire to exercise, even if today you don't.
- Getting mad at yourself for not wanting to do the things necessary to change the behaviors that are not in line with a healthy soul? Trust and try to believe or imagine that your next thoughts will be positive, even if you might doubt yourself in this moment.

Remember that we can focus too much on the goal—the outcome we want—rather than the process of achieving that goal. In life, just as in a tough race, sometimes it's about putting one foot in front of the other to get to the finish line. You have to put all your energy and strength in those single steps forward, rather than waste precious energy on thinking about being done. But the faith you have in yourself and the fact that you know you will get to the finish no matter how far in the distance it may seem is enough to carry you through.

Jilt Jealousy

Being jealous of another person's body, fitness, job, success, position in society, character, or personal possessions can hold you back from getting there yourself. An athlete who is jealous of another's accomplishments often becomes impatient, which more often than not tricks him into pushing harder than is wise, which is a certain recipe for failing to ever get there. Remember nature's timeline? Being jealous of another person's good qualities distracts us from using the ones that we have. Jealousy can erode self-confidence and keep us from using the gifts that come naturally for us.

Solution: Find Your Unique Beauty

Recognizing that every person is beautiful and valuable in his or her own way shifts jealousy. Each person is special and unique, like the colors of flowers. A blue flower isn't more beautiful than a red flower; a red flower isn't more valuable than a white flower. And a flower is no more or less important than a tree or a blade of grass. This is a positive way you can view your own body and soul. You are a unique being with a distinct purpose. Let your heart sing with its own true and unique beauty.

Filling Emotional Holes with the Light of the Fire

Fear, anger, and jealousy affect different areas of your body. In the Huichol tradition, it is said that anger affects the stomach, fear affects the throat (which can cause a weakness in the voice), and jealousy and greed affect the heart. Fortunately, there is a wonderful exercise that balances the effects of these emotions and brings power to your life.

- To begin, anchor yourself by sitting down on the ground outside, or a floor inside. You can also use a chair if needed. Feel your connection to Mother Earth beneath you (whether you are inside or outside) by visualizing a cord of energy that goes from the bottom of your back (your coccyx) down into the earth.

- Place a candle in front of you, or, if you are outside and the situation permits, build a fire. Now look at the flame with both your eyes and your heart. Imagine your heart opening as a flower blossoms in the spring and takes the light in. Seeing with the heart can be the same as having a feeling or emotion. Try to feel a kinship with "Grandfather Fire."

- If you are feeling jealous, breathe in the light of the fire. Just breath normally. Imagine the light of Grandfather Fire coming into your heart.

- If you are feeling angry, breathe in the light of the fire. Visualize it coming into your stomach.

- If you are fearful, breathe in the light of the fire. Visualize it coming into your throat.

- Continue to focus on the fire and visualizing yourself breathing in the light of the flame for about five minutes. It will have an astounding effect on the region of your body and the emotion that is associated with it, whether it's anger affecting your stomach, fear affecting your throat, or jealousy affecting your heart. ❀

Find Strength in the Nerika

Overcoming negative emotions and feeling joy happens by uniting your body and soul. Scientific research proves this concept. Illustrating the positive impact of this union, many research studies have specifically shown that when people exercise regularly they experience an increase in self-esteem and have a more positive attitude about life. The reverse of this has also been indicated by studies which link depression, stress, and low self-esteem to inhibited athletic performance.

Your body and soul are bonded together with love to form one integrated entity. By loving your body for all that it is and all that it may not be, and by taking care of it the best you can, your soul knows happiness. When your heart is happy about life and feels empowered through living, your body has energy and feels taken care of. Having good thoughts for the possibility of the changes you are working toward in your body and soul happens by feeling and experiencing this unity.

How to Give Away Negativity

Often getting out the door to do a workout or take a walk can be stopped cold when we doubt ourselves and lack confidence. You start thinking to yourself that it's not worth the time, you have too much else to do, you're too tired, etc. The list of excuses is endless. If you doubt yourself long enough, a general mood of negativity will take over. If working out has become a challenge, or doing a walking exercise for the soul seems fruitless, or any other time when facing something challenging, you can give away any negativity that might be holding you back. This important process helps you to get rid of doubts. It will help you have positive thoughts that encourage action and help you follow through on your intentions. Here is an exercise to help you do this.

- Begin by standing outside in front of a fire or candle with a small piece of wood in your hand. Feel yourself connected to the earth, the sky, and everything around you. We are all naturally connected to everything around us, and so it is good to be consciously aware of this connection. You may concentrate or meditate on this connection.
- The Huichols say to clean yourself off. Brush the wood over the top of your head, over your heart, and over your stomach.
- Place the wood onto the fire. In this way the wood is helping to give you a spiritual cleaning. If you are using a candle you can use a very small stick or a toothpick.
- Let go of the negativity that may be holding you back. Imagine or visualize your negative emotions dissipating or burning away with the wood that you cleaned yourself off with. Breathe nature's positive energy into your body and soul. Visualize nature healing you in a positive way with her good energy. This is both visualization and a positive way to think or have positive affirmations of life.

The exercise has several objectives beyond helping you release negativity. First, it gives you a reason to go out into nature, to go and find a beautiful place outside where you can make a small fire (but only by following safety precautions in an area where you are allowed to do this). You don't need a bonfire; a small fire will suffice. If this is impossible to do because of the area in which you live, you can use a candle instead.

Doing this helps develop your relationship with the earth and allows you to give away a part of yourself that is holding you back from who you really are. The Huichols don't really have a word for negativity. So when they do this exercise, they refer to it as cleaning the soul.

You are undoubtedly familiar with the body part of this unity. Just look down and you will see it. But what about your soul? What is it? Where is it? As noted briefly in the first chapter, the answer is that your soul is a place within your heart. As you heart beats, your soul lives. It's a place of silence that the Huichols call the *nerika*. The nerika is a passageway that connects your being (your heart or your soul) to all of creation. It is like a window or mirror that is looking both directions at the same time: into your heart and out to the world around you. It can also be thought of as the human equivalent of the door to your house, which connects the inside of your home to the world outside. When a person stands in the doorway of their home, they are between both worlds, connected to what is going on inside the house as well as to all they can see from the doorway as they look out.

In the same way, one could say that the nerika, your soul's doorway, connects all that is going on in your heart with all that is taking place in the outer environment. It connects you, beginning with your heart, to the circle of life. It connects earth and sky. And it connects your soul and your spiritual energy to the four cardinal directions: to the east and the place of the sunrise, to the south, to the west and the place of the sunset, and to the north. Inside, you are like a miniature universe. You need an extension of that universe to connect energetically and emotionally to the literal universe—the outer world that your soul craves to unite with. The medium you can use to develop this connection is the nerika. The nerika is one of the most powerful tools you can use to unite your body and soul and overcome negativity—whatever its source.

Find the Nerika

Use this image yourself the next time you need calm or a positive thought about your life.

Begin by imagining this visionary passageway as a circle that extends out in front of you from your heart. The nerika can have an infinite number of sizes and appearances. It can be a small circle the size of a quarter, or it can be seen much larger, depending on the person, the frame of mind, and the situation. The size of the nerika might change each time you do this exercise. It is up to you.

After you have an image of the circle in your mind, envision it opening up from your heart and expanding like a spiral, getting larger and larger, to encompass all of creation. The expansiveness of the nerika can eventually connect you to anything in the universe through a tunnel or passageway.

Negative thoughts are not who you really are. Once you have the image of the nerika, imagine anything negative or disturbing floating away outside of yourself. Inside the nerika or circle of life is calmness, a place of rejuvenation and awareness. 🔯

The nerika is the calm center that great athletes call on when they need endurance, when they have to make the big play, or when they have to rise up and come from behind in a race. When you look to that nerika, you are imagining a doorway that connects your desires and wishes with the outer world where you are trying to create your reality. It is a place that you go into spiritually, a special place of introspection where you can find your inherent joy and happiness.

Finding your nerika starts by focusing on the love of the universe. Love is behind everything that was created in the world and in the universe. When you focus on that feeling of love, you can feel the calm and the joy that is there. This is not to say that you won't still have times when you get upset in your daily life. We all do. But at these times of stress, you can recall the nerika and its calm to help keep you going.

The Huichols are able to remain calm no matter how chaotic or negative a situation might seem by going into the nerika, the visionary doorway. As we said, this is a visual link that you can imagine as a circle that exists just in front of you at the heart. This is your heart's connection to the outer world, a doorway that links you to energy and all of creation.

Visualize your attention in the center of this sacred circle. Doing this quiets the mind so you can focus on the positive, rather than the negative aspects of life and of your environment. By placing yourself in this doorway of happiness, you are able to rediscover your original enthusiasm for everything around you and inside of you. This is where you are—you have found that original spark that set you on your journey to begin with.

KEY #4:

Reconnect with the Natural World

Good health for body and soul are much easier to maintain than they are to achieve in the first place. Stress (outer influences) and the three negative emotions of fear, jealousy, and anger (inner influences) have the potential to creep in and keep us from being in good health. This is most easily combated with a good dose of preventative tactics. Why wait until stress or negativity hits to become strong to deal with it? Who would choose to have depression set in and then fix it when it's possible to fortify yourself against feeling this way in the first place? Why not take a few steps to have joy, feel energized, be balanced, and experience peace? All people in every culture around the globe have a yearning to simply feel good about life, to have a sense that in the big picture everything is as it should be.

One big endeavor that we will focus on in upcoming chapters to bring these feelings is exercise. It changes our physical appearance and makes us stronger, which adds to a positive sense of self-esteem. It enhances the quality of sleep we get, reduces stress, improves our outlook on life, and reverses the negative effects of old, unhealthy lifestyle choices—all of which brings back hope for changes in body and soul.

However, as we all know, there's a limit to the magic exercise can work. It won't counterbalance every job stress, time demand, or deadline. A long run won't raise your kids or pay your bills. Even with a fitness program to help relieve stress, daily existence can seem like nothing more than ongoing crisis management. Then negative emotions sneak in as we become disconnected from the sources of good feelings in our lives.

Over time these demands can take people another step away from the connections that are preventative medicine for keeping us physically and emotionally healthy, even during the tough times. We end up distancing ourselves from our friends and family. We disconnect not only from our neighbors and our communities, but also from our environment and our natural surroundings.

Today people often live relatively isolated lives, which is ironic given that never before has technology—like computers, cell phones, video, etc.—allowed people to have so much access to one another. But the reality is that people have far less personal contact. In addition, because of city life, we are no longer as connected to the natural world as our ancestors were just a few generations ago. We can even forget that the earth exists below us as we sit at a desk many stories high in an office building. But an essential key to having a Fit Soul and a Fit Body is to foster our connections to family, to our environment, and to all that lives on the earth. This is important preventative medicine for maintaining the balance and health of body and soul, whether you are an athlete, a diplomat, or a student. Recent studies on health and longevity support this simple idea, showing that individuals who interact regularly with a community of people, who work and walk on the earth, have the highest probability of living long lives devoid of physical and emotional illnesses.

We might try to bring back a good feeling about our life by seeing the latest hit movie, buying a new car, or maybe absorbing our attention with a new piece of high-tech equipment. And while doing these things can bring us a certain sense of fulfillment, we can't buy a new car every day. A hectically paced life has moved people in the modern world away from taking the time to witness simple ongoing events in nature that can sustain a feeling of well-being deep in our souls. This is how we are set up to stay healthy and strong, to have good thoughts and find the energy for the important things in life.

How to Foster a Connection with the Natural World

The lifestyles of our ancestors afforded them a greater connection with the earth, and they received significant solace from witnessing and feeling connected to simple yet profound occurrences in nature. A sunrise or a sunset, with all its wonderful color, brought happiness to their hearts as it does to each of us when we witness this dramatic show of nature. Working intimately with the earth for food fostered an understanding of the sacredness of all life, which helped our ancestors feel they were a part of something bigger than their own life and existence. Who hasn't been touched by a rose that blooms in a garden or the trees coming to life in springtime? These are the experiences that can give a human being the sense that everything is as it should be, which makes our soul happy.

Just like our ancient bodies that respond positively to exercises that mirror the steadily moving lifestyle of the past, our soul responds and is nourished best through experiencing the events of life that were taking place in ancient times. Feeling, experiencing, and connecting with these same events as they take place today is the currency that makes our souls rich.

The Huichols give us a window into how we can do this in our own life. They center their existence on having a deep gratitude for just being alive, even with the challenges it can present. Happiness is their starting point, not the end result. They also recognize that the strength of their bodies is directly connected to their soul's bond to their communities, to all that lives on the earth, and to the earth itself. For a Huichol, freedom comes from having these connections. And when our souls feel free, our bodies stand tall, reflecting power and joy. Every rhythm in life is united by a strong desire to develop these strengths, both of body and of soul.

A Huichol fosters these connections by recognizing first and foremost that a human being's body is directly connected to the body of Mother Earth. We are an extension of her body, just like a tree or a flower is. This is not just a metaphor. It is something both real and at the same time magical. The earth sustains us, helps us to survive, and nourishes us with the power of love. In the modern world we foster love for our family and friends as a way to feel good and survive.

Brant's First Connections to Body and Soul

Having grown up in the modern world, I had to reconnect these two aspects of my life—body and soul—as a very first step during my apprenticeship in Mexico. Don José would send me off into the mountains of the Sierra Madre, telling me to find a place where I felt well and could quiet my mind. Don José instructed me to feel the land around in every part of my being. He told me to breathe the essence of the land into my soul and into my heart.

Sustainable soul fitness started by extending this concept of giving and receiving love to include the love of the earth, which, according to Huichol tradition, is just as alive as the mother who gives life and love to her newborn child. This is part of Huichol teaching that can give meaning to your life.

You probably experienced this feeling of connecting to the earth the first time you saw a tall mountain peak, a vast forest, or an open hillside with the grasses swaying in the wind. You might have had that feeling of "WOW!" Whether you knew it in that moment or not, your soul and your heart were feeling love both for that place and from that place. And in that moment, all the problems, stresses, and worries of life disappeared. This is a beginning experience of a Fit Soul. It is one way to fill your physical body up with energy, life force, or kupuri.

Once a person has felt a connection with the earth, it becomes something important and powerful in their life. Why else do we dream of that wondrous vacation as we flip through a travel magazine with photos showing magnificent places in nature? These are the places where your soul can easily feel bonded to Mother Earth. Your soul has a special connection to her that is felt with the emotion of love. We might forget this when we are walking through a department store or waiting in a subway, but we should try not to, because remembering to feel love or good positive feelings for the earth strengthens your soul and gives you courage.

The techniques in this section will help you make a deliberate connection with the earth and will become as important for helping you to maintain a Fit Soul and a Fit Body as your time spent sweating in the health club. You gradually become a complete and a whole person by doing these exercises. Consciously connecting to all that is around you, to the four directions or the four elements, affects your body, heart, and soul in a positive way and helps strengthen your life's journey.

Maybe not every step along the way is going to be an ecstatic reflection of the love of the earth, but little by little your body will reflect the joy and happiness of the earth in your heart. You can apply this development of joy and happiness to your daily life so that you can have a great workout, a great run, a great walk, or a great experience sitting on the earth because you will be connected. You will feel part of all life. You become plugged into the energy that sustains all living organisms here on this planet.

With the advent of the modern world and the industrial revolution, our bodies have become out of sync with this ancient connection to our earth. It can become a goal of yours to rediscover this point of connection, to balance your body through your workouts and through your approach to life, and to connect your body with the earth. Making this connection, having a sense that you and the earth have a special relationship, has helped children with Attention Deficit/Hyperactivity Disorder reduce their medication needs, lessened depression, and been shown to increase the brain's capacity to function intellectually. This is just as important to developing the fitness of your body as your physical workouts.

You can make this connection to the earth and to all of life in a very simple way. Go for a walk and visualize an umbilical cord coming from the end of your spine and going down into the earth. This is a very real energy cord that always anchors you and always connects you to the earth. Then, from your heart, imagine or feel another cord extending out from your soul, a cord that connects you with everything that you see in front of you. By doing this you are connected to the earth from the front and from the back. And in making this conscious connection to the earth from your body and your soul, you are also connected to all that lives on this earth. It is very simple, yet powerful.

Making this connection is the same as when you make eye contact with another person. You are making a cord of connection. This is a physical as well as mental connection that happens simply by looking at someone. It's like when you "feel" someone looking at you, even though your back is turned. Subconsciously we feel an energy connection. Imagine then how powerful it can be to consciously make this connection with the earth.

Here are four more exercises you can do to fortify your body and soul. They act as preventative medicine that shields you against whatever may hold you back in life. They are especially helpful when you feel your life needs a jump-start. You can also do them regularly as a way to keep yourself charged up. Why wait until life takes you off track to get back on?

Connect with Mother Earth's Love

Exercises for developing a Fit Soul are just as important as those for developing a Fit Body. Your body responds positively when you exercise it. It changes form, becoming stronger and often leaner. Your soul responds positively when you connect it to nature. It becomes stronger, happier, more at peace.

No matter where you are on your journey, one emotion that strengthens your soul is love. Mother Earth's power is love—perhaps the strongest power of all—and you are an extension of her body and her power of love. Here is another exercise to help you bring this into your being and into your life.

- Wherever you are, start by walking. It can be in a city, the country, or in the wilderness. Walk in a place where you can feel at peace with yourself. As you do this, try to stop your thoughts and your internal dialogue. Try to go to a place between two thoughts. Walk slowly, putting one foot in front of the other.
- Quiet your mind. With each step you take, visualize Mother Earth's love coming into your body through your feet and traveling up to your heart. Fill your heart with her love. Let the love of Mother Earth dissolve any problems you may have. Do this for fifteen to twenty minutes. Feel that special connection to Mother Earth. Feel her love flowing into your body and empower yourself with it.

You can also do this exercise as you run. For at least part of your run, try to do what we just described. Visualize the love of Mother Earth coming into your being with each jogging step. Feel that love coming into your body with each running step you take upon her. It may sound simple, and it is. But try it. It is also powerful.

Becoming Centered between Earth and Sky

Being comfortable in our bodies and having peace in our souls no matter where we go on the earth, no matter what is going on outside of us, regardless of the endeavor we are engaged in, is related to experiencing our proper place in this universe, directly between earth and sky. Here is a practice that gives you a sense of being in the middle, between these two great forces in nature. It is a practice for your inner environment as well as your outer world. It balances your soul and helps you become a part of balancing the power of earth and sky. It is perfect to do while you are on a walk in nature, or anytime that you are outside. Walking is the most natural way to go to a place in nature where you can get away from modern life and connect with the power that has existed there for millennia.

You can do this practice any time you feel your life needs balancing. Perhaps demands on your time, emotional strain, or a lack of exercise have you feeling like the different aspects of your being are not in harmony. This exercise will help bring your soul back to a feeling of centeredness or balance, and will allow you to become a part of the world in which you live.

- Sit or lie down on the ground. Feel your connection to the sun and the earth.
- Visualize the light of the sun coming down through the top of your head. Feel it throughout your body and in your heart. Concentrate on this image.
- Now imagine that light going down into Mother Earth. Feel connected to both the light and the earth.
- Feel your connection to the earth. Draw the love of Mother Earth up into your heart and throughout your body. Imagine this as a natural happening in this process of feeling connected to the love of Mother Earth.
- Send that love to Father Sun. Feel your connection to all life.

KEY #5:

Honor Yourself

Sometimes our need to change either body or soul is motivated not so much by an inherent desire to build good health but rather as a way to make up for something we feel we lack, such as the simple need to love ourselves. It can cause people to overtrain or adopt lifestyle choices that are destructive, and can result in low self-confidence. We lose a sense that our life—our body and soul—is worth honoring with positive action, with exercise and good thoughts, good food and good friends.

Self-love is the most immediate tool you can use to fortify yourself against negative emotions like fear or self-doubt. It doesn't involve anyone but you. It has nothing to do with what others think about you. Self-love transforms need into peace. It's a feeling that comes by telling yourself: "I'm okay even with the things I may still want to change in the future, and even with the problems I may have right now." Just as your body needs vitamins and minerals for good health, your soul needs love. This helps honor you.

Begin by feeding your soul with the memory of who you are beyond your physical body. This starts with remembering how you are connected to your environment and to all that lives on the earth. Honoring the sacredness of your own life by feeding yourself thoughts of self-love fills your soul with the nourishment that sustains it and makes life worth really living. Having self-love connects you with the desire to honor your body with good health and exercise. Self-love connects you with the desire to eat nourishing foods. Self-love makes it possible to give love to your family, friends, and to complete the circle of life by giving love to Mother Earth.

Find Strength in Self-Love

With the simple thought "I can," you'll achieve self-confidence. It gives you strength and peace by washing away doubt and allowing you to trust yourself. "I can" is a statement of confidence in life itself. "I can" is fuel for the soul that sparks the desire to work out. "I can" dissipates the fear of failure. "I can" turns a boring workout into something empowering and adds strength to your life. A positive image of being strong brings resiliency and confidence in yourself, in your own inner power, your ability to function in the world, and your connection to the world of spirit. Self-confidence brings you well-being.

Beat Boredom

The more self-love you have, the greater your ability to beat boredom, draw strength from your community, become your own inspiration, and ultimately honor yourself as much as you can. The modern world is littered with those who have succeeded in changing their body and soul for a brief period, yet have been unable to find the consistent inspiration they need to make these changes a lifelong affair. The reasons why they weren't able to keep going are common. Some lament their lack of motivation, while others say they just got bored and lost interest. Less common are the people who have almost too much motivation for their journey. We want you to be one of these success stories.

Boredom dulls the soul and takes away enthusiasm for what comes next. Being bored is not the state your soul craves, nor is it the attitude your body searches for to drive its actions in the world. Undoubtedly, learning how to transform boredom is something we can all benefit from.

Find What's New in the Old

One of the most important things you can do to overcome boredom is to find what's new in the old. A Huichol perspective is to always witness life, be grateful for it, and honor the simplest gifts it brings, like waking up each morning to be alive for another day. With this as a focus, there is very little room for boredom because each moment brings the chance to see something new, even in the things one has done over and over, like working out or doing a spiritual practice, or harvesting corn or making tortillas, something that is done over and over every day of our lives.

Finding the New in Old Workout Routines

If workout boredom has you down, try some of these ideas to help bring back the motivation:

- Change your workout course. The new view will stimulate your soul while it gives your body a new stimulus.
- Do the familiar course in the opposite direction. The undulations and scenery will come at different times, which challenges your expectations and keeps your mind active.
- Find workout partners. Community is very important in helping keep workouts (and life) interesting.
- Pick a different sport or activity. Variety brings new challenges for your mind and body.
- Work out at a different time of day. Every hour of the day has its own unique quality. This is particularly noticeable when you work out outdoors: what may seem boring in the middle of the day can be magical at sunrise or sunset.
- Take a workout trip to a wildly beautiful place in nature. This may not be a daily possibility, but occasionally take a weekend, pack up the training gear, and head somewhere that inspires your soul. ✿

Embrace the Power of Repetition

Repetition is a part of all that takes place in nature, from the cycles of the seasons to how a human being is able to lose weight and learn to live with positive thoughts. The sun rises and sets over and over, without boredom. The seasons have changed year after year for millennia, yet they never tire of this repetition. Boredom has no place to live when you strive to make yourself a mirror of this. When you recognize the important role repetition plays in your life, it can be empowering. Just as the ancient ancestors did in Huichol cosmology, you recreate your world over and over again with your actions and thoughts.

You work out over and over again to maintain the health of your body. Lifting weights over and over is what builds muscle. Learning a new language by practicing it over and over keeps the brain young. Reading throughout life can also maintain mental alertness. Doing aerobic exercise day after day is what melts off unwanted pounds, makes the entire cardiovascular system healthy, and can lead to Ironman victories. You do the same in other areas of your life, too. You work the same hours to build your career. You meet up with friends and loved ones over and over to preserve and nurture those bonds. You spend and save money over and over again to reach certain financial goals. There are rituals in every aspect of our lives—from the moment we wake up and brush our teeth (a repeated habit) to the minute we put our heads down on the pillow at night (another repeated habit).

Anything you do over and over can be looked at either as something boring or as one of the greatest duties that you have in life. You do the spiritual exercises over and over again to empower your soul, help create beauty, and cleanse what is no longer needed in your life. The act of shifting one's perspective from boring to fulfilling is an exercise that can be practiced any time the mood is less than enthusiastic for your journey.

Overcoming a Boredom of Spirit

Your soul may need a spark to keep from getting bored on the road to becoming who you want to be. This can be simpler than you think if you use a few of the following tips:

- Ask yourself what is important in your life. If the answer is something you are not doing enough of, you may want time to make some changes in how you spend your time.
- Readjust your expectations. There are times when you might think you should have already attained a particular achievement, yet find that you are still struggling to achieve your goal. Instead of becoming bored or impatient with your journey, make whatever it is you are doing at that moment the priority instead of the end result. Let your present actions inspire you, and find fulfillment in them.

- Suffer with dignity. Not everything in life will be easy. Sometimes you have to suffer through something boring or uncomfortable. During these times, find the place of calm inside your soul that can be at peace anywhere on this planet.
- Laugh. Boredom breaks down with laughter. It may not change your outer world, but it will help your soul feel good.
- Give thanks. Your soul is free to live unbounded when it is grateful. And if you are alive, there is always at least that one thing to be grateful for. What bores the soul may still be there, but your soul hopefully won't be affected by it.
- Stop over-thinking. Stop allowing boredom to sneak into your thought process. It is your mind that causes boredom. Your soul is busy taking in all the beautiful impressions that surround you.

Find Strength in Community

Who will your perfect partners in life be? You can have any number of partners in your journey, and some will be better suited for particular goals, such as a confidant for work-related issues, a friend for emotional concerns like alleviating depression and stress, and someone you can rely upon for challenging you physically as an exercise partner or for holding you accountable for changing addictive behavior. The ideal support system for achieving your goals of Fit Soul, Fit Body will be those people who are serious enough to commit to sowing the daily kernels of corn that will bring success (the daily workouts, the daily steps to gradually improve your character and your ways of approaching the world), but who also feel joy being part of each of those steps and can be happy and light in the midst of their commitment.

Maintaining the motivation you need to make the changes you desire is made more effective with individuals or groups that support those endeavors. You can gain additional strength to maintain motivation through your connection to like-minded people with a common goal. One study showed that the biggest influencing factor that helped people work out was being in a city or environment where others were also working out. Anyone who has worked out at a busy health club knows this.

You can draw strength from others—your family, friends, co-workers, and workout partners—to help you in your own life. Community is an important part of all cultures. It is one of the three core aspects of healing in the world of the Huichol. One aspect is the healing of our self, doing what it takes in our life to find our health or personal healing. The second aspect is the healing of our community, bringing harmony and truth to our interactions and connections with each other. And the third part of healing, as seen in Huichol shamanism, is the healing of all that lives on Mother Earth. This brings people together on an emotional, physical, and spiritual level. With present-day Huichols and in former times, people would hunt together, or gather herbs and fruits together. Now we do other things as community. We work together in an office and come together for sporting events. We can go on walks with our community, we can go to the fitness center with our community, and we can share food with our community as a beautiful feast or a simple meal.

In today's fast-paced world, many of us have forgotten this fundamental need we have as human beings: the need to be with other people. As we mentioned, most agree that food is something we all need. In traditional cultures around the world, an equally strong need that is acknowledged by every individual is a need to be connected to and interact with other humans. No matter where you live, no matter who you are, you still have a need for community. When you have community, you nourish your soul with one of its main nutrients. The body fills up with beans and corn; the soul does the same with community. Feed your soul with friendship. It is something we all crave. Making this connection with others has many forms in the modern world. Exercise groups, spiritual groups, and work groups can all make up parts of your community.

One of the most basic elements of connecting with others is your family. However, today many people don't have the traditional family support of the past. Fewer people are married than in the times of our ancestors. Most people do not live in the same towns where they were born or where their relatives reside. For a lot of people in the modern world, their community becomes like a family. A mentor at work can become a mother or a father. Our best friends become like brothers and sisters. Or coworkers become like uncles, aunts, or cousins. Our neighbors become like relatives.

Having good, deep connections with people brings contentment and happiness to your being. It brings you into alignment with your environment and helps make you complete as a person. The Huichols have a saying that in their community "no one stands alone." Utilize this concept for strength in your own life. So that you don't have to stand alone on your journey, build yourself a support community for all that you do. Gain strength from a personal trainer or a friend who has good knowledge about fitness to help you when you are unsure of your next step. Set up workout dates with a friend or associate. The chances of skipping a workout when you know someone is counting on you to be there is much less likely than if you are depending solely on your own motivation to make it. Engage a partner for weekly walks in nature or for watching the sunset. Use community for strength in your journey.

Mark Finds Strength in Community

For me, community was a crucial element to my strengthening program for body and soul. Believe it or not, I am actually quite a lazy person. I'm good once I get going, but getting started is one of my weakest points. This goes for everything from working out to doing exercises to heal my soul. But I had my training community that I would meet for all my key workouts. This was a support that helped me keep the consistency I needed in training.

I also had my community of support with Brant that served as inspiration to keep doing the exercises and practices that were so valuable in developing the strength of my soul. At least once a season I would go on a focused retreat to study with Brant, to immerse myself in the world of nature, to have my essence merge with the power in all life. This is the community that sustained me and helped me get past my own laziness, which can easily talk me out of doing all the things that are the most important for my life.

Become Your Own Inspiration

The exercises in this chapter are given as guidelines for making sure the foundation that you build is solid. Each one is simple, and they are all effective. Every practice is familiar to your soul. Take the time to do them. No one can do the work for you. Place yourself in front of the fire and give away negativity. Take the love of the earth into your body. Enjoy connecting to your community and your own heart through positive thoughts and actions. Use these exercises as you put your pillars of fitness and good health into place throughout life. Be steady yet flexible as you journey through the exercises. Witness the results. Become your own inspiration. You deserve it!

Chapter Four

Establish and Achieve Your Personal Goals

With trust, sincerity, and a commitment to purpose, life has meaning.

An Ironman athlete has to fall in love with repetition. How else can a person train so hard for so long and not find a way to enjoy the same training regimen? Granted, this doesn't mean I had to always take the same bike or running path, walk the same trail, or swim the same sequence of strokes over and over again. But there is a definite repeated rhythm to the act of working out; even the process of the race itself—swim, bike, run—feels very familiar when you do it more than once. There's no such thing as a run-bike-swim triathlon. And when you're in the motion of each of these three different activities, you sense a certain beat or replication, whether it's the constant reach with the arms in the swim, the circular push-pull of the pedal, or the recurring forward movements of your feet in the run—one foot in front of the other over and over again. Huichol shamanism and tradition also embody this theme and are a model for its importance. Ceremonies, deer dances, exercises, and pilgrimages to places of power have been done over and over for millennia as a way to maintain health and balance of both people and the environment.

The exercises that Brant taught me in the previous chapter helped me to see the power in repetition, not just for my body's physical strength but also for my inner soul strength. The first time I did each of these simple practices, I had a direct experience of a better way of being. But as I repeated the exercises each time I was with Brant, my mind started to analyze and question why I had to do them again. I would think, *Is this really necessary?* But I would do them anyway because I trusted him as a great teacher.

Then it began to hit me what was happening. The first time I gave away a negative emotion, like fear, it had a particular effect that was indeed profound. The hundredth time I did so was similar, but the effect was even deeper. My soul could feel this important difference each time I did these exercises. Now I see how, just like exercises for my body, by doing them again and again, the spiritual exercises cleaned and inspired my soul. They have become as essential to nourishing my heart as food is to my body.

While you may not set your sights on winning an Ironman, finding the positive and the power in repetition can help you to achieve whatever goals you have. For example, if you simply want a fit body today but don't do anything about it the rest of the week, you can guess how effective you will be at achieving your goal. Simply reminding yourself of your goals can help avoid undue downtime in your journey. "I want to be fit. I want to be powerful. I want to be in good shape both physically and emotionally." Remember the original vision of inspiration that sparked your first workout, or the first time you saw a better you inside your soul. Repeating our goals and visions has much the same power to help us get there as does the repetition of working out. We use repetition in exercise to change our bodies. We can also use the repetition of reminding ourselves of our goals to bring us the energy and motivation we need every day. By paying attention to your goal or quest, you stop paying attention to anything that could take you off your path of completing yourself with joy and hope.

Minding Your Motivation

What makes one person's journey to vibrant health and well-being seem so effortless, but someone else's incredibly challenging, filled with land mines that keep throwing them off track? Most of us have experienced both of these worlds. Things can be going just as planned, yet in the next moment the light switches off and it becomes difficult to sustain our enthusiasm for long-term change. It would be nice if we could feel excitement and energy during every minute of the day, even during times of personal challenge. But this is about as unlikely as shedding ten pounds in a week. Don José was known for encouraging people to at least keep going, and not to give up on the task at hand.

Let's face it: Motivation goes through cycles of high and low. How we deal with the trying times can be the difference between taking a break from our routine for a week or throwing in the towel for good. In the last chapter, we explained how to get past some of the emotional and physical obstacles that can cause an about-face in our progress. Another tool for sustaining ourselves on our journey is learning to keep our sights fixed on our goals and visions no matter what the speed of our physical and spiritual development. Creating and focusing on both short- and long-term aspirations are two of the most important elements of the program.

In this chapter, you will learn steps to help you not only set your goals, but also to keep motivated to achieve them. The exercises, based on Huichol teachings, will help you connect the goals of your body with the goals of your soul, so that your body, mind, and emotions will all be working together to achieve body and soul fitness. You will learn how to:

- Set attainable goals—for both the long and short term
- Focus your attention on your goals
- Trust your ability to realize your visions
- Live what you ask for
- Find symbols of possibility

All of these steps revolve around goal-setting, which is so important that it's the next key to living a fit life.

KEY #6:

KNOW AND SET THE QUEST

The motivation and desire to achieve a Fit Body and a Fit Soul comes to us most clearly when we have an image of what we are after—a goal. The word "goal" is a modern-world version of what a Huichol uses to guide every action in his or her life. For them a goal could be called a vision, which is often an image of something yet to be created. Their visions become the force that integrates body and soul, calling each into play and helping focus their actions with purpose. An example would be the process Huichols experience when making their intricate, multicolored art. They wait for the image of a design or a story of their cosmology to come to them before making anything. They pray or ask for a dream or vision to show them what it is that they should create. Once it comes, they have their "goal" or image of what it is that they will bring into form.

Knowing what we want to create in both body and soul is the same. What fitness goal are you striving toward? What does that image look like in its finished form? What kind of a person do you want to become? What will that person embody in thoughts, actions, and emotions? What transformation of body and soul are you after? Having answers to these questions sets your intentions and helps focus your efforts. Our goals and visions are the magnets that draw us into action, and if focused on with both steadfastness and flexibility, will over time yield benefits beyond our imagination.

Setting the Big Goals

Take as much time as you need to come up with your long-term goals for body and soul. These will be the "designs" for your life worth working toward for a while, maybe even years. These should have significant personal importance. There can be uncertainty surrounding whether or not we will actually be able to complete them, but if you can, the journey and transformations you go through will become the milestones of personal accomplishment that will go down in your logbook of life. Here are a few examples of big goals, divided by those of the body and those of the soul:

Fit Body goals:

- Seeing a medical transformation at your doctor's office (lower cholesterol, lower heart rate, etc.)
- Losing significant weight and lowering your risk for diabetes

- Exercising every day
- Gaining control of negative food or nutrition habits
- Loving your body the way it is
- Looking toned and in shape
- Participating in your community's 10k charity walk/run, running your city's marathon, or competing at a high level in any sport

Fit Soul visions:

- Becoming a more loving and kind person
- Ridding yourself of overwhelming negative thoughts
- Building self-confidence
- Healing emotional wounds from the past
- Living a life of no regrets
- Finding peace and fulfillment in all that you do
- Going deep on a spiritual path

All of these examples are worthy goals for body and soul. Every one of them can be challenging yet exciting to shoot for. Completing them will require both body and soul working together as a united whole. Each can bring joy, power, and a deep sense of accomplishment along the way, especially if one's starting point is quite far from the end goal. **What are your life visions and goals for body and soul?**

Reality Check

Goals related purely to your physical body are often quite definable. Running a marathon is very specific. It will require covering 26.2 miles all in one shot. Losing fifty pounds is very clear, and there will be no doubt when this goal has been met. Because of the concrete nature of Fit Body goals, it's relatively easy to assess whether or not the goal is within the realm of reason, as well as to track your progress along the way to getting there. The most common "unreality" about Fit Body goals is the timeline that people set for accomplishing them. It would be an unrealistic goal for a person to expect to lose fifty pounds in one month. However, doing it at a safe rate of one to two pounds per week and taking up to a year is achievable and sustainable. The only requirement for accomplishing the big Fit Body goals is to start with what you feel is a realistic timeline, but then be willing to adjust it based on the actual rate of progress . . . being steady, yet flexible.

Goals related to your inner soul or spirit are usually less measurable. Becoming a more loving person is subjective. It's tough to chart whether or not one has been successful at changing negative thoughts into positive ones. Often knowing a Fit Soul goal has been fulfilled only happens after the change has occurred. Staying on track with transformations of the soul are most easily seen by reflecting on our day-to-day actions. "Was I kind in my interaction with a family member today? Did I stop and change a limiting thought into a supportive one when I felt doubt yesterday afternoon?" Make working toward changes of your soul a daily practice. This is one way to redesign who we are from the inside out. These become the reality checks that give good feedback on the Fit Soul journey.

Short-Term Goals

Every vision comes to fruition one step at a time. For an athlete, thousands of hours of training, doing the same things over and over and over, go into creating the ideal moments of perfection called victory. And the greatest victory of all is using one's ultimate vision or goal as the motivation to win the small victories called day-to-day work. "What can I do today to develop my body, to make it stronger and healthier?"

The long-term goals are the image of where we want to end up. Short-term goals are more like the building blocks and signposts along the way, or the steering wheel keeping us on the right road. Here are a few ideas of short-term goals for body and soul that can improve your chances of long-term change:

- Pick one limiting thought you frequently tell yourself. Every time you catch yourself thinking along this line, stop for a minute and remind yourself to live with the opposite quality that is a positive. Replace "I can't" with "I can." Make that

The Pace of Weight Loss

For losing weight, the equation just in terms of exercise looks something like this: A pound of fat has about 3,500 calories stored up in it. For the average-sized person to move their body one mile, they burn about 100 calories. Walking or jogging that mile burns the same amount of calories; walking just takes longer.

So to burn a pound of fat through exercise, an individual would have to cover approximately thirty-five miles. That math is pretty eye-opening. To lose a pound a week from exercise alone, a person would have to run or walk five miles per day every day of the week. Of course, by moderating food intake, the amount of exercise can be reduced, but this is the reality of weight loss if looked at strictly through exercise.

For a professional cyclist who can burn over 4,000 calories in one long ride, losing body fat is not a problem. For someone walking two to three miles a day, the amount of time needed to burn off that same one pound of fat can be up to ten days. In the end both people can lose the same amount, but it will take the walker longer than the professional cyclist.

The message in these two examples is that there are no shortcuts to weight loss, and unless a person's timeline for change is reflective of his or her approach, more likely than not the pounds will stay and disappointment might be the victor. A long-term approach that becomes a permanent lifestyle change is a key to success in this area, with a combination of diet and exercise that will trim the waistline over time.

shift over and over until you begin to see more and more time pass between moments where a negative image comes up.

- Take at least one moment every day to charge up your soul with a quality in nature that was around long before the modern world.
- Add in one extra workout per week for the next six weeks.
- Up the length of your longest exercise by a sizable enough chunk that your body knows it has done something special.

- Cut out one food that you know stands in the way of your desired changes. Keep it out of the house and out of your life for six weeks. This can go hand in hand with the added workout.
- Laugh. Have you laughed today? Did you laugh yesterday? The Huichols say laughter breaks down self-importance. When we can laugh with others or at ourselves, it can take the pressure off that feeling that something is wrong unless everything is perfect. And with that, gratitude ensues. What better short-term goal is there than to feel gratitude along the way to achieving our big dreams?

A Great Goal for the Body: Motivate Yourself Out the Door

Sometimes the biggest obstacle to working out is the inspiration just to get started. Often it is not that we dislike exercise, but rather that we dislike the idea of getting going. Yet once we do, more often than not we really enjoy working out. Simply beginning your workout is one of the most important short-term goals. Once you start your exercise program, other goals, such as the intensity or duration of the workout, will become your focus. But you cannot begin to achieve those if you never get started. Here are a few tips that can help you get going:

- Plan to do your workouts at a time that has the highest probability that you will actually do them. Some people need to exercise in the morning, others at night. Whenever is best for you, in terms of free time, energy, and ability to get the exercise done, make that the committed time for your training.
- Engage a friend. It's easy to skip a workout when it's just you that will be doing it. It's less likely to be a failed attempt if you know your friend is waiting at the trailhead for the walk.
- Be prepared to work out whenever the opportunity arises. If you don't know when you might have time to exercise, have your workout clothes with you at all times. This can mean having a gym bag with your gear in the trunk of your car so

when that long meeting gets cancelled late in the day, you can quickly switch gears and get in a workout, whatever kind it may be.

- Commit to doing the first five minutes of your planned workout. There may be a valid reason why you are resisting an upcoming workout. You could be too tired to exercise and really need the rest. But often, once you start the workout, whatever was holding you back dissipates and you feel the joy of finally doing the exercise. Commit yourself to exercising long enough to at least break a small sweat, even if it's only for five or ten minutes. At that point, the joy may have come back and you can give yourself a big pat on the back for creating another fitness success!

Identifying Your Purpose

Energy for developing your soul becomes available when the changes you are working for have meaning, when you recall the image of the self you are striving to become. Clarity of vision gives purpose, which dissolves the boundaries that can exist when life is not lived with reason behind it. It transforms what might be a boring or redundant task into something joyous and worthwhile. This is exemplified in the way the Huichols approach their sacred Dance of the Deer ceremonies. Some of these go on for long periods and can last day and night for days at a time. It can seem endless, just as a workout can seem endless. To dance almost continuously with just short breaks throughout the night is something that clearly takes a lot of energy. But Huichols are able to go beyond normal limits because there is purpose in the dance.

The Dance of the Deer is the Huichols' most sacred dance. It has been practiced for millennia to celebrate light and the birth of the sun. It is usually done outside and has many different levels. One part of the dance is very sacred and spiritual. You are dancing your prayers, hopes, and wishes onto the altar of Mother Earth as a way to bring her love into your heart and into your being to make you happy. You are dancing for good crops, or for a good life for you and your family. You dance for all people, all of life, all of creation. You also do it to find your essence or your soul in that special silence that exists between two heartbeats, by entering a state of awareness where you feel your connection to the sacredness of all life.

With each step of the dance upon Mother Earth, the Huichols are trying to think good thoughts, just as you can do with the rhythm created by your feet during a walk or a run. There is a continuous steady beat of the feet upon the earth, like a heartbeat that is connected to the heartbeat of the earth and to the sacred drum. The Huichols are praying *for* the earth and *to* the earth, dancing their prayers into her. They dance to celebrate their lives and the light that is in all of creation, and to be in alignment with the sunrise and the sunset, both of which are happy times for the world to be celebrated.

They do it with the purpose of celebrating the birth of a new day and the four seasons. Their dance helps open the hearts of the people and transform their souls with the rhythms and sounds of the shaman's chants. This simple act brings their bodies into alignment and harmony with their souls, with the essence of their being. All this happens as you dance in a circle around the sacred fire, one foot in front of the other, on the sacred altar of Mother Earth. Then in the morning as the sun comes up, they feel like they have completed something that has real meaning.

They also have folk dances, which are accompanied by folk songs that are beautiful expressions of the joy and happiness they feel to be living breathing human beings. The Huichols dance the rhythms that are being played into the earth. Just by dancing upon this beautiful altar they create happiness, joy, and a feeling of well-being. They go back and forth between a heightened state of awareness and just being happy and celebrating life, laughing even. If somebody trips or something like that happens, it is usually an occasion for a burst of laughter.

Brant's Experience with Don José—Getting to the Heart of Purpose and Intention

I had a funny experience once when I saw a Huichol dancer bump into Don José's chair. In order to not hurt Don José, the person tumbled off to the side and a burst of laughter erupted through the village as the people watched this scene unfold. It added to the dimension of the Dance of the Deer and the whole concept of dancing for life, dancing for joy, dancing for celebration. This ancient form of movement brings the community together and transforms an ordinary steady step into a celebration of happiness because it is done with purpose. The Huichols say this is what the universe likes to see. This is what we like to do here on the earth. And this is one of the best things that we can do. They ask innocently: Why else are we here?

Intention is what sets their dance apart as a sacred act and makes it a completely joyous experience for their community. You can experience the same happiness when working out if you do it with the same purpose, with the thought of giving thanks for your life and all life, giving thanks that you are alive as you exercise. We see a similar sense of community at a running race, for example. Thousands of people come together to run on Mother Earth with purpose, some just to finish and others to test their limits. This transforms the boundary of tiredness, boredom, or lack of interest by turning others' and your actions into a powerful community of support, a prayer or positive affirmation, and a celebration of life.

Another experience I had that brought the idea of intention and purpose to the forefront of my mind was when I brought Don José to America with me for about a month, just after I finished my apprenticeship. We were staying in Bodega, California, near where I had started teaching a Wednesday night class about the Huichol tradition. It was held in the building where they filmed the movie *The Birds*. I was also scheduled to go to Oregon to teach my very first seminar, and I told him it was going to be a twelve-hour drive.

The morning we were set to leave, he announced, "I don't want to go! You go without me."

I said, "Grandfather, I can't go without you."

"Don't worry about me," he said. "I'll just walk home."

Keep in mind we were in Northern California and he lived near Guadalajara, Mexico, thousands of miles to the south. I said, "Grandfather, I can't leave you, and furthermore, how are you going to find your way home?"

"What do you think I am, an idiot?" he asked me. "I know how to get home. You just walk south and when you get to San Blas [in Mexico], you turn left and go up into the Sierra Madres. That's our sacred land, Grandmother Ocean, and our sacred area. I can find my way back."

I tried to explain to him how you organize a seminar, and that people would assume we were going to be there, which was hard to explain to someone from a culture like his. He didn't respond.

The countdown to the workshop had begun, but of course I couldn't leave him. We sat there together in almost complete silence for a few hours. Then just as suddenly as he had pronounced he was not going, he stood up and said, "All right. Let's go!"

We jumped in the car and were off. The first part of the drive passed without either of us speaking. I didn't dare give him an opening to change his mind again. But after a while I asked, "Grandfather, what was that all about?" It was so uncharacteristic of Don José. He was someone whose word I could always count on. He had never done anything like that before. When he said he would do something, he always did it.

He answered back, "Well, I was testing you to see if you were going to chase the fame and fortune of workshops and seminars and leave me to fend for myself. You passed the test, Grandson, and now we are going."

With my intention and purpose proven, we had one of the most beautiful seminars that I have ever done.

Focus Your Attention on Your Goals

Knowing your direction, your goals, is precious. The next step is to pay attention to this knowledge and not just forget about your aspirations. An athlete is always trying to remember what his or her goals are during the day-to-day training that could otherwise become a quagmire of repetitiveness. A Huichol in the Sierra Madre Mountains in Mexico also pays attention to a quest or a goal in order to make it happen, whether the goal is to finish a piece of fine art that came to them in a dream or plant a hillside with corn, one kernel at a time, until the job is done.

Using focus to successfully pay attention to your goals can be accomplished in several ways:

- **Set aside time to reflect on your goals**. One of the best times to do this is when you are trying to decide what your next step or workout should be. The choices you come up with could be quite different if the end goal is what influences the decision rather than your immediate mood or life constraint.
- **Appreciate the importance of your daily actions**. Each positive shift your soul makes in the world, even if it seems small, is another step you are taking toward achieving your Fit Soul goals.
- **Turn your attention away from negative thoughts**. These limit our soul's ability to function well in life. They also hold us back from believing in our ability to make the transformations we are after in both body and soul. Focusing on a positive outcome can be done in many ways. First, as we just said, keep remembering your goals and what is important about achieving them. Continually rededicate yourself to not only appreciating your daily actions, but to actually taking one step and then the next as a safeguard against becoming paralyzed into inaction by thoughts of possible failure or boredom or feeling like it's just not worth it. See challenge as a normal part of life. It makes success worthwhile.
- **Have structure in your plan**. Many people respond well to structure. If winging it does not keep you on track for having a Fit Soul and Fit Body, give it form. Make a schedule of your workouts and your personal goals each week. Hold yourself accountable to them. This creates clear, short-term, week-by-week goals. Make it a priority to change your body and soul. Life fills whatever space we leave empty. By paying attention to the health of these essential elements of who you are as a human being, there is no space for laziness, and no volume to the thoughts that tell us we are too busy to do something about them or that the goals are not important. You may also find it helpful to keep a journal that records your action steps, how you're feeling each day, and anything else that comes to mind and that you think will help you in

your journey. Journaling is a great way to stay attuned to your goals, and to look back at earlier times from which to draw inspiration and strength.

Paying attention brings joy and happiness to life because you are working toward completing something. It may sound like a paradox, but every beginning point is also an ending point. By beginning a workout, you end being inactive. By focusing on connecting to the beauty in life, you stop being disconnected from it. By following a program for your body, you stop ignoring your health. By following your heart's desire, you end your search for what your heart is seeking. Paying attention to having a Fit Body and a Fit Soul makes it possible.

Appreciate the Importance of Your Movements

During your next outdoor workout (walking, jogging, hiking) start with most of your attention on the mechanics of the exercise. For example, if you are walking or running, notice how your body responds when you use different stride rates and lengths:

- Watch your heart rate.
- Take note of when or if you start to sweat.
- Make a mental note of your perceived level of exertion at this point.
- See how undulations in the terrain affect all of these things.

These are some of the mechanical aspects that go on during a workout, which can give important feedback on your Fit Body progress. With increased fitness, your pace will get faster for a given heart rate, and it can feel easier to go fast at a higher fitness level than it did going slower with less fitness. What once may have felt like mountains will become manageable hills. This will help create a distinct contrast to what comes next.

Now, turn your attention from what your body is experiencing and onto your surrounding environment. Think about where a Huichol might be focusing his attention as he moves. His attention would be focused on drawing in the love of Mother Earth through his feet. With his heart he would be feeling a connection to the life that surrounds him. Now remember that Mother Earth lies below you. If even for just a moment you can feel her love, or have gratitude for your life as you look around you, you have made strides toward a Fit Body and Fit Soul connection. In those moments you are free of what bothers you, of any doubt or distraction that could deter you from your goals, and of all the things that normally consume a modern person's attention. You have become a human battery getting plugged into nature's socket to be charged up and healed.

In Chapter 3 we went over two great exercises that can help you plug into life and the appreciation this can give. One was Connect with Mother Earth's Love (page 74) and the other was Becoming Centered between Earth and Sky (page 75). Both of these tools can be used in the middle of a workout or in the middle of a crisis as a way to bring a sense of happiness, clarity, and hope to the situation. The outer world may not have changed by doing these two exercises, but your internal environment can become more positive and powerful.

Recharge Your Enthusiasm

When the joy and motivation for your program is high, it's rarely even a question whether or not you are working successfully toward your goals. At other times, because of life circumstances, there can be the need to refocus your body and soul to stay on track with your dreams.

We can use exercises of the soul to refresh and enliven the body whenever we feel the need. If you find that even after getting out the door for your workouts you still lack enthusiasm for what you are doing, reduce the amount of time you spend on the upcoming days' physical activity and instead do some of the exercises for the soul that can help bring back a positive attitude.

Revisit some of the Huichol-inspired exercises from Chapter 3 as a way to shift your focus away from some of the negative thoughts that can creep in when we feel unmotivated. For one week, practice each one of these exercises for twenty to thirty minutes:

- Connect with Mother Earth's Love, page 74
- Give Away Negativity, page 66

- Be Fearless in the Face of Your Fears, page 60
- Transforming Anger to Trust, page 63
- Filling Emotional Holes with the Light of the Fire, page 64

Allow Exercise to Recharge Your Soul

Exercise can also help when life overpowers your ability to have a positive soul, when you get bogged down with pressure and joy is replaced with hopelessness. The next chapter will help you to establish a conditioning program attuned to your lifestyle. Don't let your fitness program become a burden—use light exercise, particularly in times of stress, as a means to relaxation and renewed energy. At times, working out can be used as medicine for the soul more than as a way to build the health of the body. When you feel inhibited from achieving your goals due to time restraints, stress, or fatigue, employ these Fit Body tips to mend your soul:

- If you can't find enough time for a long or intense workout, walk, walk, walk. Take even a few minutes several times a day to go outside and disconnect with whatever is weighing on your soul and just walk on Mother Earth. You can do this during coffee breaks, between clients, or after dropping the kids at school before launching into the chores that will take up your day.
- If your soul feels beat up, be good to yourself with your exercise. Recharge with an easier training session than planned. Make your workout into something soothing by reducing the intensity, cutting back on the length, finding a friend to come with you, or picking a route that has scenery that soothes your soul.
- Remember, if you are bored or unenthusiastic about your regular workout, find a new road or trail, or try an entirely new activity. Refreshing your soul can come when your immediate environment is also fresh. This can also signal to your soul that whatever rut it might be in can also be changed for the better.

These exercises are quite effective for helping you shift your focus back to having a feeling of trust in your ability to achieve your goals. Keep in mind that the aim of each of these exercises is to help you feel motivated again. Keep walking, for example, until your problems and worries are replaced with joy and hope. Sit in front of a candle or fire until you begin to feel the three negative emotions (fear, anger, and jealousy) shift and diminish. Becoming an expert at this simple exercise—shifting your focus—can be one of the most important skills you have to help you achieve your goals.

Trust in Your Ability to Accomplish Your Goals

There are many feelings a human being can have that motivate you to take action. Motivation might come from a negative emotion, such as fear, anger, jealousy, or insecurity. Or it may come from a more positive feeling, such as joy. When we feel joy or excitement for a task, it becomes something we look forward to doing. When we feel joy for a workout, we can hardly wait until time frees up to go do it. When we feel joy or motivation for life, we want to make the time to absorb the beauty all around us. Feeling joy for a Fit Soul and Fit Body inherently comes when you feel you are going to get something out of it that betters your life. Why go to the gym over and over if you don't feel it will transform your body? Why immerse yourself in the study of a certain subject if you don't think it's possible to find any satisfaction by using it professionally in a fulfilling career? Why spend the time to take in the beauty of a sunset if you don't think it will make your soul feel better?

We feel enlivened when we are connected to the possibility of being happier, more positive, and more able to deal with the world. Seeing where you want to go on your journey of body and soul creates trust that it will happen. It sparks you to begin this journey. Trust brings that powerful motivator we call joy into play by building a bridge between where you are right now and where you want to end up.

Ancient peoples such as the Huichols trusted in the spirit of nature when they saw how it sustained all life over time. They experienced firsthand how rain and light mix with earth and air to nourish all that grows on the earth. The Huichols see this as something both ordinary and exceptional at the same time, and it enables them to trust in the natural world. Trust creates the hope of possibility, of something fulfilling and satisfying. Start by trusting that you can indeed create a magical state of being that is both natural and impressive. By this the Huichols mean that you can accomplish whatever goals you want and at the same time feel satisfied with yourself. You can trust your heart's desires or emotional desires and make it a reality as you develop your personal goals. This belief and trust helps you to love the process of developing a Fit Soul and a Fit Body.

Huichol Wisdom: Breathing in Joy

Some of the greatest insights into life come when you are still, just breathing in the air that surrounds you. The next time you feel you are lacking a sense of trust in your ability to accomplish a task that lies in front of you, stop everything and just sit for a moment and focus on your breath. Use the cycle and rhythm of air going in and out of your body to visualize joy or hope coming into your being. Allow this joy to bring you a sense of calm. Let it wash away whatever is holding you back at that moment. Then when you have this feeling inside, begin again with whatever it is that you may have had trouble undertaking.

Each Fit Soul and Fit Body exercise that you do is an affirmation of the possibility of achieving your goals. If you can't see the changes you desire happening at a particular moment, trust that in time you will. Acknowledge that you do indeed want to have vibrant health from the inside out. In the shamanic tradition, it is said that to want or ask for something is an affirmation of trust and hope that it is possible. Having trust in your ongoing ability to transform yourself allows you to experience your world in a way that is like being held safely in the hands of life or the universe itself.

Focusing on Trust

If we need renewed enthusiasm for the road ahead, whether it's for the steps necessary to become more positive in life or for another workout, first remember and believe in your original goal or dream. As we said earlier in this chapter, remembering your original inspiration helps shift your focus away from the negative and toward rediscovering beauty, your good spirit, your good self, and all the great qualities of your soul. Next, bring in the concept of trust. It is one of the most powerful motivators we can call upon for help. Trust in your ability to make the changes that were inspiring at the beginning of your journey. Here is a way to use trust to refresh motivation.

Remember that feeling of intrigue that powered the first days of shifting your habits. Remind yourself what originally inspired you to undertake a particular goal. *I want to run a 10k. I want to end my unhealthy lifestyle habits. I want to find satisfaction in my job. I want to live a more balanced life.*

Next, remind yourself what moved you to truly take the steps to transform your soul. Recall the hope for a better life that inspired you to attempt a more fulfilling existence. These memories are a bridge that brings back inspiration and allows your dreams to move toward reality.

Let these positive thoughts affect your actions. Let them spark your original enthusiasm and then continue on your journey of transformation of body and soul.

Finally, visualize your journey taking place with these good thoughts. Visualizing your success over and over again allows you to stay involved with your original enthusiasm. Use this any time there is a lull in your motivation for a workout or a race, or a hesitation to let go of unwanted qualities of the soul.

KEY #7:

LIVE WHAT YOU ASK FOR

Truly being free to achieve your Fit Soul and Fit Body goals is only possible when you live what you ask for. Asking for a healthy soul but engaging in friendships that are volatile or unsupportive can create a barrier to finding this peace. Asking to win a race but giving up halfway through does not accomplish this goal. You wouldn't want to ask for a fit body and then eat all your meals at an ice cream shop. Sure, ice cream is fine once in a while, but living your dreams requires following through with your original intentions. Take in foods that nourish your body (see Chapter 6) and the positive energies that feed your soul. Live with the thoughts and actions that empower you, not ones that weaken you. Surround yourself with people who share your values. Focus on having a positive attitude, seeking the support of friends, deepening healthy relationships with your community and environment, and always looking to find your higher self within. These are positive actions you can take that will help you live what you ask for.

Sometimes we would rather do what is easy and abandon our goals when living what we ask for gets tough. It can require a certain amount of tenacity to win the small battles of will that allow us to do what we know is the better choice (sticking with our program). Huichol cosmology is filled with stories that reflect this need. One is how the sun goes into the underworld at night and battles with demons in order to be reborn at dawn into freedom. This can be a mirror for your own life. Perhaps you are also battling with your own negative desires. We all have these battles. For some, it may be succumbing to eating too much rather than being empowered by eating the right amount for our bodies. Others might regularly come up with reasons why they can't sign up for a course that addresses a hidden passion and that could lead them to finding their true calling in their daily work. Living what you ask for means doing what we have said earlier in this chapter, which is to first remember your goals, then use that vision to transmute negative thoughts into positive desires and actions. Then you become free to live without the limits of inconsistency.

The Bigger the Quest, the Tougher the Test

Living what you ask for starts by acknowledging that there will almost always be tests along the way to living a powerful life filled with possibility. These tests are just barometers to see if you are indeed willing to live what you are asking for, to see if you are willing to hold on no matter what to your vision for life is. And as you have probably experienced, the bigger the quest, the tougher the test is likely to be. Asking to lose five pounds is not going to present the same challenge as asking to lose fifty. Transforming a way of living that you've practiced all your life will be tougher than changing a lifestyle that was adopted just recently.

This is fine. Plan for it. Transforming body and soul does not have to take place overnight. Remember you have your whole life to live a strategy that is fulfilling to you. Time is a great healer and a great teacher. To overcome difficult tests that might confront us, we can sometimes trick ourselves into believing the test might not be so challenging. As Don José used to say, "If you're not happy, make believe that you are and you might trick yourself into becoming happy." This is simple advice that can be applied to the most intense challenges along the way. Everything from the toughest hurdles in fitness to the personal changes that seem to be taking an eternity can be brought a step closer with this simple thought.

Expect the tests. Remember the tools that can help get past challenges. Here's a quick recap of the ones from this chapter:

- Motivate yourself out the door.
- Remember the purpose of your goals.
- Pay attention to your goals.
- Recharge your enthusiasm.
- Trust in your ability to fulfill your dreams and visions.
- And most importantly (hence the key), remember to **live what you ask for**.

The barriers that hold you back from living your vision dissolve when you go through the tests. They are not barriers to fulfilling your aspiration of Fit Soul, Fit Body; they are tests, and all tests are finite. They are simply pivotal moments asking you to live your dreams. Face the test of the quest, no matter how difficult or how frequent. You will make it through. Call out to your higher self for what you need to go through and beyond the test. Examples of affirmations you can say to yourself: *Give me the strength I need to keep going. Help me to find my way through this test. Help me to learn what I need to from this so I can go on. I'm trying, so help me.*

Find Symbols of Possibility

You can work with symbols for the healing of body, heart, and spirit as a way to find strength in living a life without boundaries. Positive symbols allow for a human being to feel that he or she has a purpose, and a reason to be here. Our goals can give us that feeling of purpose. Positive symbols are concepts, ideas, or models of reality that you can follow to help bring possibility into your life. Boundaries melt when we feel something is possible to accomplish. In the modern world there are many tangible objects that become symbols of possibility. A gold medal, for example, conjures up images of an athlete reaching for possibility through the years, and then finally making her moment of perfection something the world can see.

In your own life, a powerful symbol can be to simply visualize having success, not only in a particular field of work, but also at maintaining a healthy soul and a healthy body. These last two images are very powerful manifestations of what happens when you have positive thoughts. Keep those images of body and soul that mean something to you alive as symbols of possibility for today, and then tomorrow, as symbols of success. Let them become symbols for your further success in the years to come, for your completing your life in a positive fashion. Become your own living symbol or representation of having a Fit Soul and Fit Body.

When you notice a Fit Body change, it becomes a living symbol of your success. Each moment that the wonder of nature makes your soul blossom with good feelings is a symbol of your success. They represent your capability to transform, change, and move forward through life. Hold on to them and use these symbols when you need to renew your hope and see a more clear vision of possibility.

Having a goal, image, dream, or vision of where you want to go and what you want to accomplish sparks the actions that will lead you there. Every successful business is guided by visions laid out by its leaders. All athletes have a big vision of success that they strive for, which motivates them each and every day in their training. The

Huichols use visions and dreams just the same as a guiding force for their actions in everyday life. Use the visions or goals you came up with in the beginning of this chapter as a magnet drawing you into action. Remember them when you need help.

Take challenge as something natural that will ultimately empower you along your journey to the essence of a Fit Body. This journey begins with a request to life:

> Give me what sustains me.
> Help me to find what I need to keep going in my life, to
>   find what propels me and gives me energy.
> Bring purpose to my actions so they have meaning to my
>   soul. This is sustained through my personal symbols
>   of success that come from my visions of possibility.
> I'm asking for clarity of vision so I can see where to go,
>   what I need to do. With this image, help me to live
>   what it will take to get there.
> Help me to trust in my own abilities.
> Help me to live what I have asked for.
> Bring joy and clarity to my journey.

This is what helps bring a Fit Soul together with a Fit Body. ✿

Chapter Five
Find Your Conditioning Program

Physical fitness allows us to activate the good health, good thoughts, and positive sense of self that is coded inside our genetics just waiting to come out.

You don't have to be un-athletic to feel intimidated at a gym. Before I turned thirty-three, I was able to compete in triathlons on par with the best in the world without lifting anything heavier than my bike when I put it in the back of my car. But at that age something started to change in my body. I noticed that I just didn't have the same strength I used to when climbing hills on my bike. I couldn't find the speed on the run. My shoulders fatigued quicker in the pool. And my speed of recovery was slowing. It seemed like I was working out harder, but my fitness was going in the opposite direction. I knew I had to hit the gym.

So I went down to the health club near my house. It was one of those places where the grunting was so loud it would drown out the music. I stopped at the door. I looked at the bodies of the people working out in there. Then I looked at mine. I froze. I felt like I was a different species. There I was, the Ironman Champion, intimidated to go into the gym and lift weights because my body didn't match what I saw through the door to the weight room.

I was supposed to be an expert at getting in shape. I had swim, bike, and run down pretty good. But I couldn't have told you the difference between a lat pull-down and a side lateral raise to save my life. I needed some help. So I contacted a local woman who was an expert in the field of personal training. She led me through an entire season of strength training, which brought back the muscle I was losing and enabled me to get back to the level of training that was slipping away so quickly. Now, almost two decades later, I still do the same program that I started at age thirty-three. In this chapter, you'll learn a program you can do routinely to preserve your muscle strength and maximize your agility and power. No matter where you're starting from—or how intimated you may feel at the thought of stepping into a gym—you can make vast improvements with just a few simple exercises. And you can even create your own personal gym at home without ever having to join a gym or spend lots of money.

Something else that changed my conditioning for the better was learning how to use a heart rate monitor. I learned this trick earlier in my career—before the wins started coming at the Ironman triathlon—and you can benefit tremendously from learning how to use one, too, even if your physical feats are easy walks. We'll teach you how to use one properly in this chapter, and show you how to find your target heart rate, which may be different from what you previously thought. I owe a great deal of my wins to learning how to keep my heart rate in check and literally slow down to get faster! (You'll understand what this means shortly.)

Before I started using a heart rate monitor, my usual training program entailed working out as hard as I could. I thought if I didn't train fast, how would I ever become fast? But my race results were abysmal. I was always tired, was often sick, and never had a placing in a race that matched what I thought I should have been able to do based on all those long hard workouts in practice.

The first time I used a heart rate monitor in training was eye-opening. I had to add more than three minutes per mile to my running pace just to keep under my target heart rate. In other words, *I had to slow down*. And going up hills I had to walk slowly to prevent my heart rate from skyrocketing. My pace was so slow at this heart rate that if I ran at that speed in the races, I would not even have been able to place in the over-fifty-year-old category. Imagine that . . .

and talk about self-doubt! I was in my twenties, and thought I was a world-class athlete! The reality was that my physical fitness could not even match that of people twice my age. But over time, I saw how moderating my heart rate was giving me steady improvement. I became healthier, my energy and enthusiasm became consistent instead of fluctuating up and down, and my race fitness improved vastly. And perhaps the most important aspect of this type of training was that I finally started to enjoy what I was doing! That is our goal for you, too. By beginning this Fit Soul, Fit Body program and lifestyle, you are making a conscious choice: a choice to live a better, more fulfilling, and accomplished life. We can't think of a more profound decision to make, and we're excited for you and the improved health that awaits you.

So with that in mind, let's turn to the secrets of finding a balanced fitness program. It's essential to finding a life of health and happiness.

Create a Balanced Fitness Program

More than 90 percent of the people who start a high-intensity fitness program are likely to quit after three months. Many of us have been there, dedicating ourselves to fitness with our New Year's resolution. But we often undertake a training program that is too vigorous or doesn't successfully address our goals, and then we throw in the workout towel after only a couple of months. As you develop your program, it is just as important to create a routine that doesn't exhaust your body and end up adding unnecessary physical or mental stress as it is to make sure enough effort is put into your training to actual stimulate your body to respond with improved fitness, health, and strength. We're going to help you do that.

Remember, finding a life of balance must include physical health. If you haven't been active in a while, that's okay. This program contains ideas for those just starting out, or those coming back to a more active life after being relatively sedentary. This is when you will watch and feel the elements of both Fit Soul and Fit Body coalesce. It's a magical alchemy for discovering the balance in life that so many wrongly think is mythical. It's not. And you will discover that when you find balance in your exercise program, it will be easier to find balance in other aspects of your life—at home, at work, and in your relationships with colleagues, friends, and loved ones.

The Huichols find this balance, as did all of our ancestors before the modern age, in their active lives. They carry heavy loads of wood and water (similar to strength-training workouts), walk for hours to and from the cornfields (similar to cardiovascular workouts), and dance to celebrate their lives during sacred ceremonies (a social outlet that encourages the connection to other people). In their world, having a Fit Body is a natural result of living a life that is intimately tied to their natural surroundings. Remember, physical strength also means developing a relationship between your physical body and the body of Mother Earth.

Unfortunately for many of us, our surroundings consist of a computer screen, a television set, and a car that takes us between the two. Even the way some of us exercise is different from the steady walk of someone living in an indigenous society. We may gravitate toward short-burst, high-intensity workouts either by ourselves or in a group setting. Exercising consistently at high intensity, however, pushes the body beyond what it is designed to absorb, and will prohibit real long-term fitness.

One reason for this is that high-intensity training turns off the internal flames that burn the body fat most people are trying to get rid of. Another effect is that if you work out at high-intensity levels all the time, you will continually be tapping into that part of your genetic makeup that is reserved for dealing with highly stressful situations—the adrenal system. This system is not designed to be activated on a regular basis. If you overuse it, you can feel depleted and tired. Your energy reserves will start to feel low. And when this happens, you know the result . . . it gets harder and harder to get up for your workouts.

Too much adrenal stimulation through high-end exercise depresses the immune system and leads to getting sick more frequently. And even if you don't get physically sick, constantly using your "fight or flight" response depresses your ability to have the good feelings about life that your soul so desperately craves. This can lead to irritability and depression, which inhibits your ability to deal with normal, everyday life. It also increases the chance of having a heart attack and heart disease. None of these consequences fit the objectives of a program designed to give you sustainable body fitness and a sense of well-being.

High-intensity workouts have their place in training as a way to refine a good base of fitness and fine-tune your body for competition. This comes in the form of speed work that we will talk about in a moment. It is also the key element in most fast-result training programs because high intensity does get quick results, at least in the short term of up to a few months. However, it's not a sustainable approach to fitness, no matter what fitness goals you have, from weight loss to becoming a world-class athlete. To ensure that you do not overstress your body, it will be important to engage in a fitness program that incorporates exercises of varying types—both aerobic and strength training—and monitor the intensity at which you are working out to be sure you are in an effective training zone. Which is exactly what this chapter is going to help you achieve. It will be your roadmap for finding a comprehensive and balanced fitness program attuned to your body and fitness level. We call it the Fit Body Conditioning Program, and after a brief overview of the program, plus ideas on exercises and secrets to reaping the most benefits from both cardiovascular and strength training work, we'll help you put together your own personal program based on your fitness levels and goals.

Be Smart at the Start

If you want or require additional help in tailoring this program to your body, especially if you have any special health concerns or needs, please speak with your doctor or medical specialist. Your personal health practitioner can provide extra guidance and individual support. We also encourage you to keep your doctor in the loop if you plan to commence an exercise program and have not been active in a while. Everyone's response to this program and results will be different.

Prelude to the Fit Body Conditioning Program

The Fit Body Conditioning Program is a great way for workout novices to get started on the road to peak physical conditioning, but the program is also ideal for those who are looking to achieve a higher level of conditioning and athleticism with their current exercise or sports program. Because everyone has their own workout goals and experience, we have tailored the Fit Body tools for three levels of fitness:

1. **The Adaptation Program** is ideal for those just starting out or those who are ready to get back into exercising after a long break.

2. **The Core Program** can help bring a more efficient structure and focus to those who already engage in a regular workout routine at a moderate and consistent level.

3. **The Performance Program** incorporates tools that will bring a competitive edge to anyone committed to a high level of fitness and athletic performance.

Each of these programs will be described in detail, with easy-to-read charts, starting on page 144. The spectrum sounds broad, but we will show you that building a strong base of body fitness is similar for just about any sport. Certainly every activity requires sport-specific skills to excel, but achieving a core of strength and the conditioning needed for those finer skills is what we will address. You will be led through the nuts and bolts of building up your cardiovascular system, the lungs of your fitness program. In addition, we will provide you with a total body strength-training program that is simple to follow yet extremely effective in helping you gain added lean muscle so that all activity becomes easier. These two elements of Fit Body Conditioning—cardiovascular and strength training—are important no matter what your sport of choice is, and regardless of your current level of fitness.

The third and distinctly unique piece of the Fit Body program will be incorporating Fit Soul exercises in a way that will connect your efforts by uniting body and soul. No fitness program is sustainable if body and soul are not aligned.

In keeping with the goals of Fit Soul, Fit Body, you will see how your fitness program can be designed to become something that is sustainable for life—the variety of activity levels we will suggest keep boredom from being a limiting factor. The concept of sustainability is what sets the Fit Body Conditioning Program apart from other approaches to fitness. Many workout programs get immediate results by challenging the body to an extreme level, sacrificing a person's ability to keep the program going over time. Remember your long-term goals from the last chapter? Achieving goals over time and maintaining results is what characterizes Fit Body Conditioning.

If you are a strength- or speed-sport athlete, you might ask why you need aerobic cardiovascular conditioning. And likewise, many people who like aerobic sports, such as running or swimming, forgo strength training, believing it unnecessary. These are both important misconceptions. Having a balance of cardiovascular and strength training in your fitness game plan will give you the dynamic edge to raise your level of fitness and performance. They are also the two pillars of success in losing weight, improving health, and increasing longevity.

Get Stronger to Reverse Aging

The secret to looking and feeling young and healthy really is exercise. And it's not something reserved for the young, or for those interested in looking like an advertisement for the perfect body. After you reach about thirty-five years of age, unless you do strength training, your body will lose at least 1 percent of its lean muscle mass each year for the rest of your life. Lean muscle mass is one of the biomarkers of a person's physiological age (as opposed to the age on your driver's license). Adding lean muscle makes you younger at any age. And, in fact, research done in the past five years indicates that exercising to preserve lean muscle mass can reverse the signs of aging at the *cellular* level.

In 2007 a team of Canadian and American researchers looked at the effects of six months of strength training in volunteers aged sixty-five and older. The researchers took small biopsies of thigh-muscle cells from the volunteers before and after the six-month period, then compared them with muscle cells from twenty-six young volunteers whose average age was twenty-two. The scientists expected to find evidence that the program improved the seniors' strength, which it did by 50 percent. But they never expected what else they witnessed: dramatic changes at the genetic level. The genetic fingerprint of those elderly volunteers who'd gone through the strength-training program was reversed, nearly matching that of younger people. In other words, their genetic profile resembled that of a younger group. The Huichols are living testament to this study. Their lifestyle naturally mirrors the Fit Body program, and the results speak volumes. Not only do they look years younger than their age, but Don José continued to carry heavy loads of firewood up a hillside until he was 108 years old!

At the beginning of the six-month period, researchers found significant differences between the older and younger participants in the active functioning of six hundred genes, which seemed to gradually work less with age. By the end of the exercise phase, the expression of a third of those genes had changed, and upon closer observation the researchers realized that the ones that changed were the genes involved in the functioning of mitochondria. Mitochondria are your cells' generators, where ATP (the energy used to fuel just about every chemical reaction in the body) gets created to process nutrients into energy. Getting these genes to become active again is proof that you are only as old as the functioning of your genes!

Here's another way to think about how important it is to preserve lean muscle mass. Starting in our thirties, we lose an average of a pound of muscle each year. One pound of muscle burns approximately 35–50 calories a day. A pound of body fat uses only 2–5 calories. Muscle burns calories; fat just stores them.

A famous twenty-year-long study conducted on marathon runners also shows the importance of strength training on the body as you age. Two groups were tracked over the twenty years of the study. Both groups trained for and ran the Boston marathon every year over that period. One group trained for the marathon by doing only running workouts and no strength training. The second group did exactly as the first group, but they added in strength training.

Both groups were measured for the amount of lean muscle mass they had and were observed to see if this amount changed over time.

The first group (running only) lost the predicted 1 percent a year over the twenty years, even though they continued to run regularly. The second group (running plus strength) maintained their lean muscle mass over the duration of the study. The conclusion was definitive: To maintain lean muscle mass, aerobic exercise alone is not enough. Strength training is the only way to ensure that at fifty you still have the muscles you had at thirty.

Are You Burning Fat or Carbs? Check Your Heart Rate

As we explained at the beginning of the chapter, checking your heart rate with a monitor during aerobic workouts helps you to stay in the right zone for optimal results. It's one way you can be sure you are working out at an effective intensity, one that allows you to build muscle and burn fat without taxing your adrenals. For the Huichols, paying attention to what your heart and body are telling you is the soul's way of finding itself at the center of wisdom. Paying attention to your heart's beating is your body's way of telling you how to work out wisely.

At low to moderate heart rates, you will be in the aerobic zone, burning mostly fat as your source of fuel for movement. As your intensity increases, there will be a point at which your body cannot keep up with your muscles' need for energy by burning fats, and it switches over to an anaerobic metabolism, in which carbohydrates become the main fuel source being tapped into for the workout. The specific heart rate at which this switch occurs—your maximum aerobic heart rate (MAHR)—is the most important number you will need to know to be able to design a sustainable workout program that will give you a Fit Body.

Know Your Number: Determine Your MAHR (Maximum Aerobic Heart Rate)

The MAHR will be different for each person and it is directly tied to your age and your level of fitness, both presently and past. You may have heard in the past that you can arrive at this number simply by subtracting your age from 220, and then using a percentage of that value. But this is not the most accurate formula. The following is a better way to figure out the key heart rate for you:

- Subtract your age from 180.
- If you have or are recovering from a major illness or an injury that lasted for more than a year, subtract 10.
- If you are sedentary or if you have colds or flu every two to three weeks, subtract 5.
- If you work out two to four days per week for about thirty minutes a workout, keep the number where it is.
- If for the past year you have consistently worked out four or more times per week for more than thirty minutes each time, or you work out a total of at least five hours a week, add 5.
- If you are over fifty-five or under twenty-five, add 5.

The resulting number is your Maximum Aerobic Heart Rate (MAHR). Training at or up to twenty beats below this heart rate will build your cardiovascular health in a very sustainable way without overtaxing your system. This is true for everyone, from the most sedentary to the top endurance athletes.

Let's take a look at an example to see how someone who is forty years old and who works out less than two days a week would determine his or her MAHR:

Start with 180, then subtract 40: 140.

Because the person works out less than two days a week, subtract 5.

This person's maximum aerobic heart rate would be 135 beats per minute.

You can see how the MAHR will vary with age and with different levels of fitness. For example, someone who is sixty years old will have a lower MAHR than someone who is twenty years old. Also, if two people are the same age, the person who is more fit will be able to work out at a higher heart rate before they make the switch from fat to carbohydrate burning.

KEY #8:

SLOW DOWN TO GET FASTER

The benefits of working out at or below your MAHR are so powerful that we're calling this a key secret to ultimate fitness (and happiness!). This sounds counterintuitive, but it works. Recall how Mark got in touch with his heart rate and from there managed to accelerate his fitness program, not to mention his actual speed.

Many people we have spoken to who stopped exercising gave the simple reason that it was too painful. That is not the goal of Fit Body Conditioning. Working out at or below your MAHR will be pleasurable to your body instead of painful or exhausting. You will be energized instead of depleted, and you will recover successfully from day to day. One of the reasons moderating your intensity level has so many positive results is that working out in the aerobic heart rate range causes the release of DHEA, which we have mentioned is responsible for giving people a positive feeling. The positive emotional state that comes from working out at the correct moderate intensity goes a long way toward reinforcing a good feeling about exercising. This is how you will be able to sustain your enthusiasm over time

Workouts that push your heart rate over the MAHR, on the other hand, call into action your fight-or-flight mechanism, which is the stress response, and is taxing to your system. This type of workout can require much more than a good night's sleep to recover from before you will feel like doing it again, due to the depleting effect of high-stress hormone levels. Over time this leads to emotional stress in addition to physical stress because it results in the release of cortisol. If activated sparingly, this hormone will make you feel superhuman. But if levels remain elevated for extended periods of time, energy levels drop, motivation disappears, concentration becomes difficult, and lean muscle gets metabolized. When interest in working out starts to wane, the culprit can almost always be traced back to a person spending too much time working out above his or her maximum aerobic heart rate.

If your goal is to change body composition and lose fat, it can be almost impossible to do if the workouts are done above your aerobic maximum number for one simple reason: **once you switch over to carbohydrate burning, you don't go back to mostly fat burning for seven to nine hours**.

How to Use a Heart Rate Monitor

The best tool for observing what the heart is doing is a simple piece of equipment that can be found at almost any sporting goods store. It is a heart rate monitor, which is basically a high-tech watch that allows you to keep an eye on your pulse moment-to-moment during exercise.

There are many varieties and levels of complexity to the heart rate monitors that are available. Some just tell your heart rate. Others store your pulse rate over the course of an entire workout and can be downloaded onto a computer later for analysis. Some even record your distance traveled and elevation gains during a workout. Most have straps that go around your chest which pick up your heart rate and transmit it to a watch on your wrist. If you have a small rib cage (most women and young people), many companies have specially designed chest straps that will conform to your body better than the standard models. Try on various models in a sporting goods store to make sure you find one that will work on your body.

Using a heart rate monitor isn't just for traditional conditioning; because it helps you determine whether your body is burning fat or carbs, it can be a wonder tool for weight loss as well. Brant found this to be true during his own journey to lose extra weight, as he explains:

The lifestyle in America is very different than the lifestyle in an agricultural society where much time is spent outside walking, gathering firewood, and growing food. Here in the modern world, with my busy schedule of teaching and traveling around the world leading retreats, little by little, over several years, I gained an extra fifty pounds. In 1997, Mark invited me to come to Hawaii when he was being inducted into the Ironman Hall of Fame. When I got to Hawaii, I was surrounded by 1,500 perfect bodies. After that experience I started working with Mark directly, using his exercise program. I began running, which now I really enjoy. We worked out in a way that was sustainable for me, using the heart rate monitor, slowing my runs down to burn the maximum amount of fat. I also began a strength-training program at the gym, and in just over six months I was able to lose the extra fifty pounds I had gained.

In the beginning, most people are surprised how easy workouts feel when they are working out below their MAHR. For people whose fat-burning systems are under-developed, even a brisk walk will take their heart rate right up to the edge of their aerobic maximum. At this speed, the pace may seem too slow to be doing any good. But it is! It just requires a little patience in the beginning until fitness catches up with our image of how fast we should be going. Try to resist the urge to go faster. If you pick up your pace, your heart rate will go over your aerobic maximum and the basis of cardiovascular fitness, the ability to burn fat, will be stopped for that workout session.

Slow Down to Get Faster in Life, Too!

The concept of slowing down to get faster has an additional meaning. Not only does this key work to optimize your physical body's capacity so it runs most efficiently, but you can also apply it to virtually every other area of your life as well. The Fit Soul exercises in particular are meant to help you slow down what could otherwise be a frantic pace for your mind, emotions, and spirit. Take, for example, the strategy of quieting the mind. When you do this during stressful moments, or when life is really testing you, you'll find that you can navigate through rough patches smoother. Problems seem less formidable and solutions become clearer. And the motivation you need to move forward and instigate positive change becomes automatic. In fact, "slow down to get faster" is a key that bridges both the Fit Soul and the Fit Body components. Whether you're feeling stressed physically or emotionally, you can always rely on this key to keep you tuned in to your needs (including the basic need to stop and take a few deep breaths) and stay poised to move forward at the right pace for hitting your goals, and for getting the results you want.

In the upcoming Fit Body program options, we'll give you ideas on incorporating Fit Soul strategies into your overall program. But before we even get to those details, let's cover your choices for finding the right elements to mix into your personalized physical program.

Ingredients in the Fit Body Recipe

Choose a Cardiovascular Exercise

Cardiovascular training can be any activity that sustains an elevated heart rate for a minimum of twenty minutes. This includes walking, jogging, swimming, and cycling outside, as well as using a Stairmaster, treadmill, rowing machine, or stationary bike indoors. If the exercise is done in the proper aerobic heart rate range, it will burn fat during the workout and also build the endurance base of aerobic fitness that will determine race results for all endurance-oriented sports. For strength sports, a moderate amount of cardiovascular activity will help increase capillary development, which helps speed the delivery of blood during exercise and nutrients during recovery. A strong aerobic system also increases cardiac output, which improves workout efficiency even in the strength moves.

Every aerobic workout makes you just a little more efficient as a fat burner, something our cave ancestors were very good at. Over time, as this ability improves, you will go faster and faster at the same heart rate. At his peak, Mark was able to run a mile in 5:20 and still keep his heart rate below his aerobic maximum of 155 beats per minute because of his efficiency at burning fat as a source of fuel, which assisted in his overall endurance and made even high-output race paces seem relatively easy.

Also over time, as your fat-burning efficiency improves, your body composition will naturally become leaner. Whether this is your goal or not, it is a nice side benefit to being aerobically fit. And it is this fitness that builds on itself over time, enabling people to sustain their effort and motivation with more steady workouts rather than the highs and lows most people experience with other programs. For endurance athletes (anyone who competes in events lasting longer than four minutes), it is the amount of aerobic training they do that will have the biggest single physiological effect on their race performance. This is contrary to what many athletes focus on, which is their anaerobic high-intensity training.

Following is a list of exercises that can help you work your aerobic system. Each one has its strengths in a Fit Body program. None are exotic, but they are all highly effective in adding to your overall health:

Walking. This universal exercise should not be discarded even by the most serious of athletes. For those simply looking for a low-impact way to move their bodies, this is one of the best. It burns approximately 100 calories per mile regardless of your pace, and can be done just about anywhere. Those who already have a rigorous exercise routine can also use walking to aid in recovery. It helps flush byproducts from training out of the muscles and helps deliver nutrients to the cells to help them rebuild, both of which are pluses for speeding muscle and tissue regeneration. This is one of the best activities to do while implementing the Fit Soul exercises (see the box on page 124 for more).

Hiking. This is an extended version of walking that can last from a few hours to several days. In addition to the cardiovascular benefits of hiking, it also affords a special chance to surround oneself with the spirit of nature. The effects of being in nature are currently under study in the modern world. The results are now supporting what shamans have said for thousands of years, which is that spending time in nature can bring balance to the body, good thoughts to the mind, and a peaceful feeling to the spirit.

Easy to Moderate Running, Cycling, or Swimming. The effort level that qualifies each of these as "easy to moderate" is any amount that targets the aerobic training range we described earlier (from twenty beats below your MAHR all the way up to it without going over). This is in contrast to the higher intensity levels that elevate your heart rate over the MAHR. Keep in mind that if you are used to training at a higher heart rate, even if it feels relatively comfortable, staying below your MAHR initially might feel like you are not getting anything out of the workout. But you are, and exercising at this intensity level can develop the part of your fitness that sustains health and performance for your entire life.

Easy to Moderate Cross-Country Skiing. This, along with snowshoeing and ice skating, can be wintertime alternatives to your summer activities.

Aqua Jogging. This requires using a jog vest designed specifically to float your body upright with your head above water. With it on, you can imitate the running motion in water. This is perfect for those who have joint pain when performing weight-bearing exercises and for those recovering from running or other impact-related lower body injuries.

Low-Impact Aerobics, Cardio Equipment, Stationary Bikes, and Treadmills. Sometimes because of weather, lack of daylight, or

Walking Is for Everyone

From the most inactive person to the fittest athlete, walking can be a potent tool to promote a life of health, balance, and well-being. You can make walking as intense as you like by adding more miles, including inclines and declines, and even adding hand-held weights. It's one of the most versatile and accessible forms of exercise there is.

Walking activates many of the fine motor-control muscles that do not get used when a person jogs or runs; this muscle development helps improve efficiency of form that cannot be attained from faster movements. It also develops the ability of the muscles to flush out byproducts of exercise quickly, which speeds recovery day to day. It burns fat, increases blood and oxygen flow to areas of the body that get less than their fair share when sitting, and can be a welcome change from what has become a largely indoor existence for most people in today's society.

If walking is your primary workout of choice, we recommend walking about three miles per day to gain the greatest improvements in health and longevity. If you are using it as a tool for recovery, even as few as five minutes a day can help speed the regeneration process.

Walking can also invigorate your soul. You've probably experienced how good you feel when you go outside and take a stroll, especially after a period of being cooped up indoors. Taking a five-minute walking break can help reset your focus and energize your spirit in the middle of a tough workday. It can help you disconnect from anything negative that might be going on in your office or home, and recharge your enthusiasm for what lies ahead. The moderate pace of walking allows you to take in impressions of the world around you, removing the boundary indoor life puts between the environment and you. This is the perfect time to stop the thinking process, which recharges an overused brain, and also to recall what is important as far as your goals and dreams.

The Huichols are a living example of a culture that walks. They walk to sacred places, to work in the cornfields, to gather firewood, and to get drinking water from sacred springs. I made numerous pilgrimages to special places in nature that took at least a day to get to and then another day to return home to the village, with a good night's recovery sleep in between! This fits our model of Fit Soul, Fit Body, health and recovery. When I brought Don José to America, one of the first things he noticed was that the people were not outside walking. Everybody was in a car. He asked where all the people were. "Don't they walk to get from one place to another?" he wondered. This type of activity is something that's important for us to do, to walk and to connect to our world through our steps in our life, which help us to find strength.

personal preference, using in-gym exercise equipment or group classes is a great alternative to doing your cardio workout outdoors.

Dance. This brings several very important elements of overall health into play. One is physical movement. A second is the development of community and doing things with other people. The third is learning new steps. All of these combined have been shown to stave off Alzheimer's, improve the effects of Parkinson's disease, and give overall gains in fitness for people who don't like traditional forms of exercise.

Gardening. One of the most common elements in longevity is working with the earth. It may not get your heart rate up very high, but the benefits are universal.

Don't Skimp on Strength Training—You Can Do This at Home

Unlike the vital elders in the Huichol culture, most people tend to lose their balance more as they age, which leads to an increased risk of injuring bones and joints. Strength training helps guard against this by activating the fast twitch muscle fibers needed to respond to sudden changes in body orientation. Doing strength training as we get older makes it much more likely that we will be able to catch ourselves before we fall.

The first step in your strength program is the most important . . . to actually start. This is much easier for some people than it is for others. There are those who absolutely love health clubs and make them almost like their second home. Others, however, have health club memberships that lie dormant simply because the gym environment is like another planet to them. If you are unfamiliar with it, this arena can initially be intimidating.

But you don't necessarily need a gym or fancy equipment to keep a solid strength-training program. As noted below, we encourage you to seek help from a personal trainer if you're unfamiliar with general strength-training exercises, but you can choose to set up a small gym at home just by purchasing free weights and resistance bands (more on this shortly). You can later add more sophisticated equipment to your home gym if you want.

Keep in mind that the benefits of strength training don't end with fat burning. We can't stress this simple fact enough: Lean muscle mass is one of the main determinants of your basic metabolic rate, so the more lean muscle mass you have, the more calories you will burn each day, regardless of your physical activity (even in your sleep!). But fat burning is just the beginning of what building the strength of your muscles does for you. Here are a few other pluses that might spark a trip to the weight room:

- Combining strength training with aerobic activity stimulates the immune system and quantifiably improves eyesight.
- Joints and tendons become more resilient, reducing the chance of injury due to repetitive use syndromes on the job.

- Maintaining muscular strength is also one of the most effective tools available to also prevent injuries in sports. Everything from ankle twists to repetitive-motion joint pain can often be avoided with proper strength training.
- Two necessary hormones for rebuilding muscles, testosterone and human growth hormone, are stimulated and released by doing weight work. Both of these help a person gain strength, make muscles and joints supple and strong, and speed recovery, all of which are benefits for anyone exercising at any level.

News flash for women afraid of "bulking up": Because women don't have the same levels of testosterone as men, women usually don't build the same kind of "bulk" that men can build. In fact, the muscle a woman builds through strength training shows up as a well-toned and sculpted body—not bulky in the least. The muscle mass will accelerate the metabolism and help you to maintain an ideal weight.

Find the Right Gym . . . Or Create One at Home

Not all health clubs are the same. If you can't see yourself sweating away surrounded by an army of 250-pound weight-hurling body builders, don't worry. Hunt around. Most health clubs cater to certain kinds of people. Some gyms are strongly oriented to women. Others have more of a family feel. And of course, some are for those who are either young or young at heart: they pump up the music while you pump the iron. The point is to find the spot where you feel comfortable and where you can get the guidance you need from the training staff if you need help. None of us was born with proper strength-training technique and knowledge. Getting help from a personal trainer, especially in the beginning, will enable you to maximize the benefits from your strength program, and will teach you proper technique to minimize the risk of injury from improper lifting style. Remember, we all start from the beginning!

Another option is to create your own personal gym at home, which we'll help you do shortly. If you are not comfortable going to a gym to have a personal trainer help you establish your routine, call a few gyms in your area and ask about trainers who can come to you.

Most will be able to help you set up a gym (or bring free weights and other portable equipment to you) and teach you the basics. If you find someone that you really enjoy working with, you just might hire him or her to come to your home on a regular basis.

The Life Strength Program

The menu of exercises you can choose from to develop your muscular strength is exhaustive. But for Fit Body Conditioning, we have narrowed the focus to the exercises that are involved with the majority of movements in life, from lifting groceries out of the car to running long distances or climbing a mountain on your next hike. The routine is designed to work all of the major muscle groups in your body in a way that gives you the maximum strength and health benefits for the amount of time you put into this aspect of your body fitness. Some weight programs isolate different parts of the body for each workout. But this is an integrated approach that takes into consideration the ancient wisdom that our body is one unit with all its functions interconnected.

As with anything, overindulgence is not wise. This definitely applies to strength training. **The Life Strength Program is most beneficial when done only two days per week with two or three recovery days separating each of the strength workouts.** For example, if you do strength training on Monday, then the second strength-training workout in that week could be as soon as Thursday but no later than Friday, which ensures that the next week's Monday lift will be separated from the previous one by two days. You can do your aerobic exercises as many days of the week as your body and lifestyle allows, as recovery from these workouts is usually accomplished with a good night's sleep. But it's different for strength workouts. For most people, doing strength training three or more days per week gives them a very diminished return on the time put in because the teardown on the muscles exceeds their ability to recover, which means they can actually end up getting *weaker* over time. It takes about two full days to recover from a good weight-training session.

Doing three or more sets on each exercise also compromises your ability to gain strength. If you are able to do three or more sets of a particular exercise, you are probably using a lighter weight than you should be, which changes your exercise to one of endurance-building rather than one that stimulates significant strength gains in the muscle.

Gym Program

There are twelve exercises in this program. Many of them employ the use of machines found in most gyms. And as we just emphasized, go through the routine two days each week, with two to three days separating each session. Never do this program on consecutive days.

Start initially with one set of 12–15 repetitions on each exercise. The amount of weight you choose should be heavy enough that by the end of the set it becomes challenging to complete the lift, but not so heavy that you are at your maximum effort. Ideally you should end the set feeling like you could have done one or possibly two more repetitions. If you feel like you could have done three or more repetitions after the end of the set, the next day you do your strength program, add additional weight in small increments relative to the overall amount being used in the exercise until you achieve the goal of being one or two reps away from your limit at the end of the last set on each exercise.

Each lift should be done to a count of two when raising the weight and a count of four when lowering it. This encourages a controlled motion during the lift as opposed to a "throwing" of the weight. Make sure that you breathe out as you lift and then breathe in as you lower the weight. Never hold your breath as you do the lift. Your muscles should be moderately sore the day after weight training. Once you reach the point where they are not sore the day after doing one set on each of the twelve exercises below, increase your workout to two sets of 12–15 repetitions.

The exercises are listed in the order that they should be done.

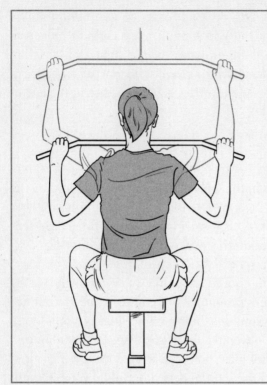

1. Lateral Pull-downs
Grasp bar with arms straight and slightly wider than shoulder width apart. Push chest forward, arch lower back. Pull bar down in front of head to shoulder level.

2. Leg Extensions
Sit on machine. Rest shin pads just above ankles. Line knee with pivot point of machine. Extend both legs fully to make a straight line.

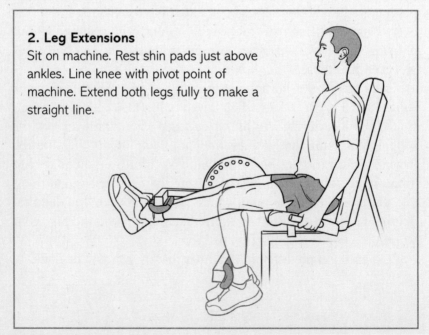

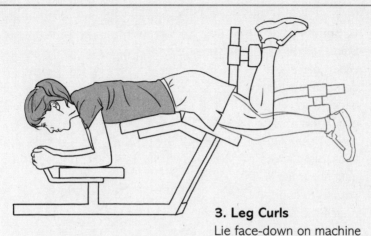

3. Leg Curls

Lie face-down on machine bench. Place leg pad just above ankles. Keep legs slightly bent. Contract fully. Keep hips on pad at all times.

4. Bench Press

Lie face-up on bench, hands slightly wider than shoulder width apart, with the bar above mid-chest. Lower bar to one inch above mid chest. Keep lower back on bench at all times.

5. Squats

Stand with legs wider than shoulders. Arch lower back. Keep weight over heels at all times. Push glutes back. Bend knees until upper leg is parallel to floor. Knees should *never* extend in front of the toes.

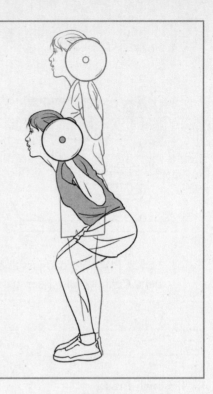

6. Inclined Press

Sit on slightly inclined bench with dumbbells in both hands at shoulder height. Extend weights overhead until they touch.

7. Forward Lunges

Stand with legs together. Rest bar comfortably on upper back. Step back, extending leg out behind. Return to standing position, dragging the toes of the extended foot on the floor on the way back up.

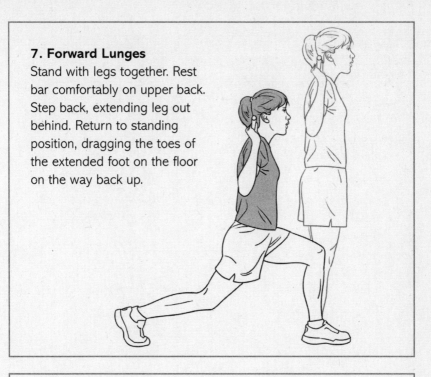

8. Side Lateral Raise

Hold a weight in each hand with elbows even with the plane of your body and slightly extended away from your torso. Extend arms out sideways, keeping elbows still in the plane of your body. Stop the lift when arms are parallel to the ground.

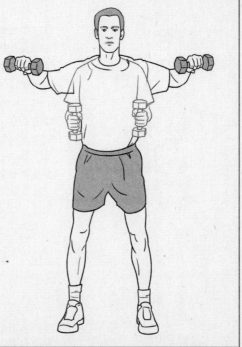

9. Calf Raises

Place one foot on a step and the other raised just slightly off the step. Hold the weight in the arm on the same side as the calf you are working. Lower heel until you feel a moderate stretch.

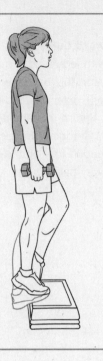

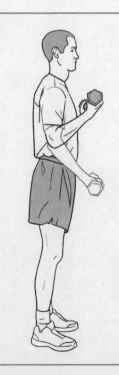

10. Bicep Curls

Start with weight lowered, elbows tight against the side of your body and arms slightly bent. Contract arms up, still supporting your weight with your biceps. Keep elbows locked tight against your side.

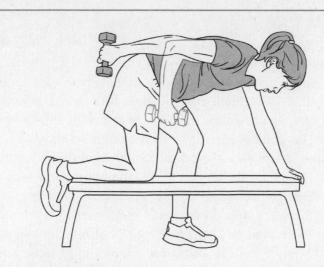

11. Tricep Extension

Place one leg on the bench, the other foot on the floor. Place the weight in the hand on the same side as the leg on the bench. Keep elbow tight against your side. Extend back fully to straight position.

12. Leg Press

Sit on the sled with your knees bent and feet roughly shoulder width apart. Extend legs fully.

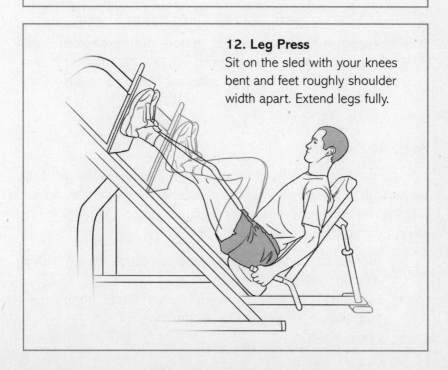

Then finish with:

- **Back Raises**: Lie on your stomach. Raise one leg and the opposite arm and hold for 15–30 seconds. Then switch and raise the other leg and opposing arm. Repeat each group twice, rest 10 seconds, then lift both arms and legs at the same time, again holding them off the ground for 15–30 seconds. This will develop the lower back muscles.
- **Sit-ups**: Sit-ups should work all four areas of the abdominal region, which are the lower, middle, and upper abs as well as the sides, or obliques, of the abdominal muscles. Life Strength sit-ups should not exceed more than 15 repetitions in any of the regions. Doing hundreds of sit-ups can give you abs of steel, but it can also cause a build up of lactic acid, which will turn off your fat-burning system and overdevelop the muscles around your diaphragm, which will cause your breathing to be shallow and restricted.
- **Modified push-ups**: Flip back over onto your stomach and do eight push-up raises. This is a regular push-up motion except that you keep your hips on the ground. This lengthens the muscles that attach to the lower back, which can get shortened by sitting for long periods of time and can cause lower back pain. Do three push-ups looking straight up, two looking left, two looking right, and then one more looking straight up again.

At-Home Program

Not everyone is able, willing, or capable of scooting off to the local health club to lift weights. However, there are ways you can mimic many of the exercises in the gym program at home with a minimum of equipment. Here is what you will need:

- Rubber stretch cords (also called resistance bands) with a door attachment
- Hand-held weights (choose various sizes, from three-pounders to roughly twenty pounds)
- Ankle weights

- A sturdy chair
- A flat thin bench (optional)

Each of these tools can help you simulate strength exercises from the gym, and you'll find them at your local sporting goods store. You can do these exercises exclusively with resistance bands or with a combination of bands and hand weights. Again, if you use weights, we recommend getting an assortment of sizes, from three pounds up. Choose what feels comfortable to grip, as many hand-held weights now come with coverings that make them easier to hold.

You can perform the following exercises as you would at a health club, at the same frequency and the same number of sets:

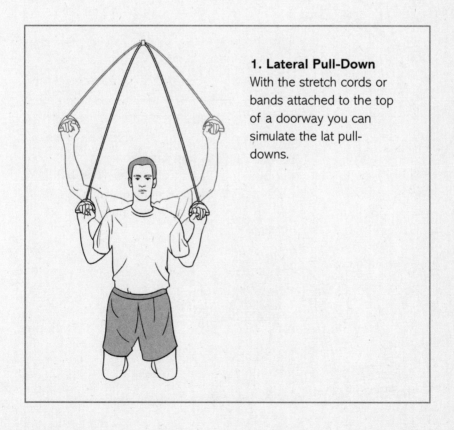

1. Lateral Pull-Down
With the stretch cords or bands attached to the top of a doorway you can simulate the lat pull-downs.

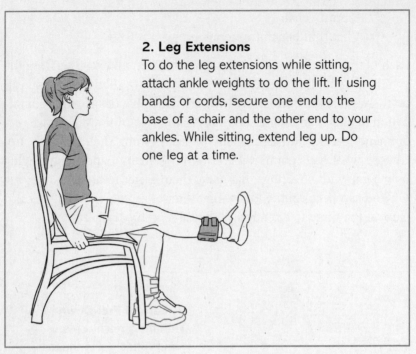

2. Leg Extensions

To do the leg extensions while sitting, attach ankle weights to do the lift. If using bands or cords, secure one end to the base of a chair and the other end to your ankles. While sitting, extend leg up. Do one leg at a time.

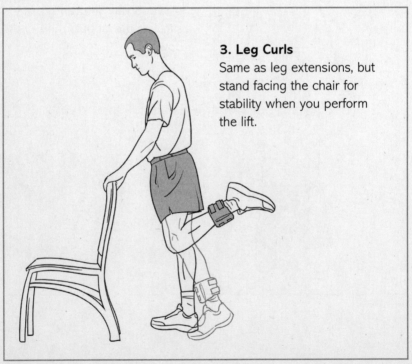

3. Leg Curls

Same as leg extensions, but stand facing the chair for stability when you perform the lift.

4. Bench Press

Use hand weights or put bands around your back. Lie flat on a bench and raise arms up straight.

5. Squats

Holding weights in your hands, go through the squat move as described in #5 above. With bands or cords, stand on them and put bands over your shoulders to create resistance during the lift.

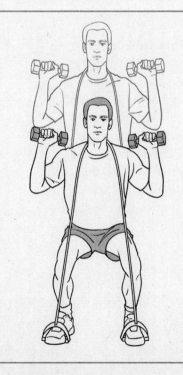

6. Inclined Press

With either a bench that can have a reclined position or by sitting reclined in a chair, hold weights in both hands or sit on cords and do lift as in #6 above.

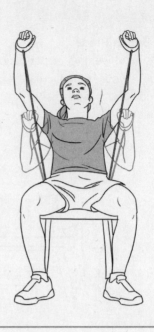

7. Forward Lunges

Stand with legs together. Rest a bar comfortably on upper back or hold dumbbells in each hand. Step back, extending leg out behind. Return to standing position, dragging the toes of the extended foot on the floor on the way back up.

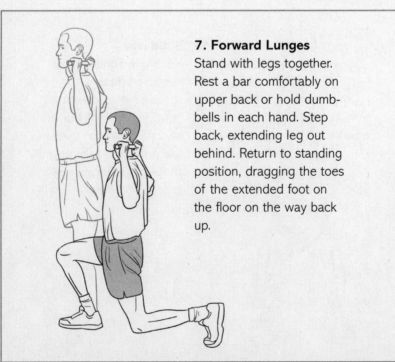

8. Side Lateral Raise

Raise weights as in #8 above, or if you use bands or cords, step on them and raise arms out to the side.

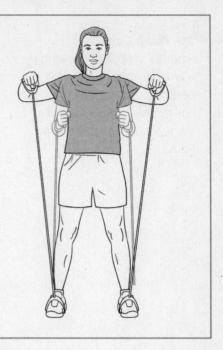

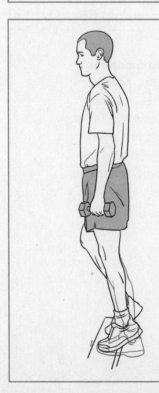

9. Calf Raises

Use a step in your house as support for your foot to lower from.

10. Bicep Curls

Same as #10 above, sitting in a chair or using a home bench. If using bands or cords, stand on one end of them, then lift one arm at a time.

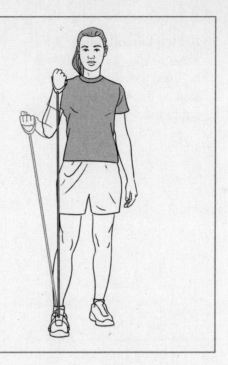

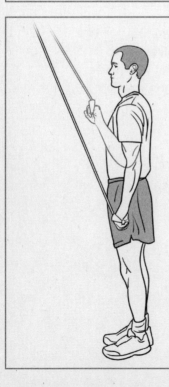

11. Tricep Extension

With weights, same as above either on home bench or on floor. If using bands, hold one end tight against your chest, then extend down with the other.

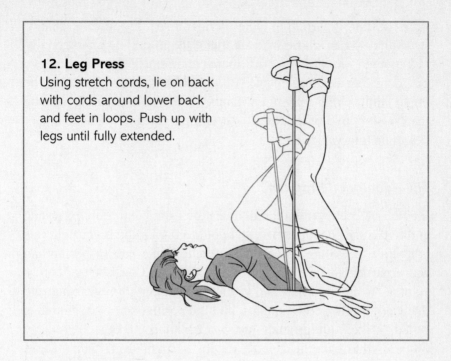

12. Leg Press
Using stretch cords, lie on back with cords around lower back and feet in loops. Push up with legs until fully extended.

Putting It All Together: The Fit Body Workouts

Figuring out how often and at what intensity you should work out depends on your goals and the level at which you are starting. The Fit Body Exercise Programs outlined below are divided into three intensity levels.

The first is **The Adaptation Program**, which is best for someone who is just starting out with a regular training routine, who has had an extended leave of absence from consistent working out, or who doesn't feel ready for either of the second two programs, but still wants to maintain a nice base of fitness.

The second is **The Core Program**, which will serve those who are regularly active but may lack a focus or structure to their program. It will also help maximize fitness and health without a significant impact on what for most is an already packed daily schedule. The Core Program can also get you ready to enjoy the excitement of doing some racing if this is one of your goals.

Our third program is **The Performance Program**, which is structured to help those who are interested in finding an extra edge at a competition. It will require more commitment than the first two programs, but will also enable you to maximize your genetics at the upper limits. This program will have more daily training volume than the first two programs as well as some extra well-placed higher heart rate interval training.

The Adaptation Program

If you have been waiting for an invitation from life to start exercising and to change some patterns that you don't like about yourself, this is it. It's time to get going! We cordially invite you to become an active participant in your improved fitness and well-being. This is your call to action! There is no better time than right now to activate the good health, good thoughts, and the positive sense of self that is coded inside your genetics just waiting to come out. Forget any obstacles that have held you back in the past. Don't worry about what might come up in the future. As the Huichols say, the only moment we know for sure is right now.

The Adaptation Program is the perfect starting point for someone who has been on the sidelines of exercise for longer than a couple of months—or maybe even your entire life. It's the entry point that will get your body used to exercising and moving. It will get your lungs breathing deeply and build your heart so it is more than a background muscle.

This program is also perfect for someone who may do a little bit of regular working out but who has never used a heart rate monitor to gauge your effort. Do your normal workouts, but use your MAHR (maximum aerobic heart rate) as the gauge for your effort instead of speed for the next six weeks and see what happens. The weeks using the monitor might require you to slow down to regulate your heart rate. Then, as your body begins to develop its aerobic engine and starts to develop more efficiency using stored body fat for fuel, you should notice a positive difference in your cardio workouts. We suggest using this schedule for at least six weeks. This will allow your body time to adapt to exercise quite nicely without risking the single biggest mistake most people make when starting out: doing too much too quickly.

The training schedule outlined in Table 5.1 burns about 1,000 calories per week through exercise. If you are trying to lose weight, cutting about 300 calories per day out of your diet along with this program will help you lose approximately one pound of fat per week! (See Chapter 6 for specific suggestions regarding your diet.) Note: we have given you a mixture of exercise options that include days doing cardio workouts in a gym as well as doing similar exercises outdoors. Feel free to adapt these options to fit where you most like to work out. We certainly recommend people exercising outdoors in nature as much as possible. However, in a city this may not be realistic. If you find that because of time constraints, weather, or personal preference that you are doing most of your training indoors, it will be even more important to balance this time with the Fit Soul practices that are the complement to your exercise program.

Fit Soul Exercises During Adaptation

We have given you many different Fit Soul exercises in the earlier chapters. Integrating them into your Fit Body Conditioning will help you sustain your enthusiasm for your exercise program and will help ensure your success by integrating the energy of your soul with the efforts of your body. Here are a few exercises we suggest using during your Adaptation Program. Choose one to do each day as a way to center your efforts in the middle of good thoughts and gratitude that you can indeed work out. The amount of time you practice them, just like exercise for the body, will vary depending on who you are. But as a minimum, you should do them long enough to feel a shift in your attitude, mind-set, thoughts, and feeling toward life.

Here are a few to choose from:

- Be Fearless in the Face of your Fears, page 60. This is great when you first start out with any form of exercise and there are the most unknowns surrounding your efforts to achieve good physical and emotional health.
- Give Away Negativity, page 66. Again, this can help to shift any doubts you have about your ability to create positive

TABLE 5.1: THE ADAPTATION PROGRAM

Day	Activity	Total Workout Time
Monday (Outdoor day)	Choose one: Walking, swimming, cycling, or other exercise where a steady pace can be set.	20 minutes
Tuesday (Indoor day)	Choose one: Exercycle, Stairmaster, elliptical trainer, treadmill.	30 minutes
	Strength training: 1 set of 12–15 repetitions on each exercise from the Life Strength Program (see page 128).	30 minutes
Wednesday (Outdoor day)	Choose one: Walking, swimming, cycling, or other exercise where a steady pace can be set. If you like, make this activity different than what you did on Monday.	30 minutes
Thursday	Off	
Friday (Indoor day)	Choose one: Exercycle, Stairmaster, elliptical trainer, treadmill.	20 minutes
	Strength training: 1 set of 12–15 repetitions on each exercise from the Life Strength Program (see page 128).	30 minutes
Saturday (Extended outdoor day)	Choose One: Hiking, power walking on trails, mountain biking, swimming, or other non–weight bearing activity.	45 minutes
Sunday	Optional activity of your choice.	30 minutes

changes and to alter any negative body image that may have held you back in the past from doing the exercise that will bring your desired results.

- Focus on Trust, page 103. You are starting out with the trust that your goals are valuable and worthy of attempting. Fortify your efforts with this exercise to trust in your ability to change over time.

The Core Program

The Core Program can build on the fitness you will gain from the Adaptation Program's exercises. It is designed around being sustainable over a long period of time as well as helping you to maximize the health benefits of working out with a minimal impact on your daily life from a scheduling perspective. You can use it for a few months as a way to get yourself ready for the Peak Performance Program, or you can use it for the rest of your life. It can get you ready to go out and enjoy a short running race, some periodic higher-intensity group training sessions, or your sport of choice. The Core Program is purely aerobic (as opposed to anaerobic), which means that it works the steady fat-burning, low-stress physiology that brings maximal health to a human being. The higher-intensity anaerobic workouts (carbohydrate burning) are part of the Performance Program. But before moving on to that, make sure that you have built your base of aerobic fitness by using the Core Program for at least two to three months.

With the schedule in Table 5.2 you will burn about 2,000 calories per week, which is what research says will give us the longest life. Note: Your actual amount will vary depending on the speed that you go during your workout. Walking for one hour in general burns about 400 calories. Jogging for one hour can burn up to twice that. We will give nutrition guidelines to complement this program in Chapter 6, which will help you tailor your food intake around this Fit Body Conditioning schedule (see page 183).

As with the Adaptation Program, we have given a mixture of outdoor and indoor exercises as a way to see how both can be done. Again, we suggest doing as much of your training outdoors as is feasible, but we know that for many reasons inside options might make up the bulk of your workout time. Just keep in mind that our genetic makeup is set up to thrive and keep us at peak levels of health in an outdoor environment. The Fit Soul practices that are incorporated into each of the three Fit Body programs will enable you to experience this.

Fit Soul Practices for the Core Program

All the Fit Soul exercises we listed for the Adaptation Program will help fortify and consolidate your efforts at any time you feel you need some extra help during the Core Program. Just like working out for the body, having a variety of practices for the soul will keep the journey fresh. Here are a few additional suggestions to draw from and use to make your program one of both Fit Body and Fit Soul:

- Connect with Mother Earth's Love, page 74. Having the power of love inside enables anything you undertake to be done with gratitude and a positive attitude. Using this not only creates an outlook on life that sustains your efforts, but also connects you to the area and environment where you train, giving you a sense of belonging and being an important part of the big picture called life.
- Filling Emotional Holes with the Light of the Fire, page 64. Sustaining the Core Program for life can require first dealing with life and then making time to train. If any of the three negative emotions—anger, jealousy, or fear—are consistently preventing you from exercising, use this practice to shift them into ones that will sustain your efforts, such as love, joy, and gratitude.
- Focus Your Attention on Your Goals, Both Body and Soul, page 96. Take some time to recall the purpose, vision, and dreams that this program is going to bring you and that sparked your interest in the beginning. This shifts your focus away from things like a short-term setback or plateau and back onto trust and enthusiasm.

TABLE 5.2: THE CORE PROGRAM

Day	Activity	Total Time
Monday (Outdoor day)	Choose one: Walking, jogging, swimming, cycling, or other aerobic activity.	45 minutes
Tuesday (Indoor day)	Choose one: Any piece of cardio equipment in the health club, low-impact aerobics, spin class (using heart rate as your guide).	45 minutes
	Strength Training: 2 sets of 12–15 repetitions of each exercise from the Life Strength Program (see page 128).	45 minutes
Wednesday (Outdoor day)	Choose one: Cycling, swimming, cross-country skiing (in winter, of course!), jogging.	60 minutes
Thursday	Off	
Friday	Your choice of activity, either indoor or outdoor.	45 minutes
	Strength Training: 2 sets of 12–15 repetitions of each exercise from the Life Strength Program (see page 128).	45 minutes
Saturday (Extended outdoor day)	Hiking, power walking, or jogging on trails or in parks, cycling, swimming, or other non–weight bearing activity.	75 minutes
Sunday	Optional: Activity of your choice or day off. If the weather is good, we suggest using an outdoor activity, especially if your job during the week requires you to be inside most of the time.	30 minutes

The Importance of Working Out Consistently

A recent study looked at the healthiest individuals in our society to see if they had any exercise traits in common. It was found that they all worked out for about one hour, five days per week, which is in line with the latest government guidelines on exercise, which recommend thirty to ninety minutes per day. This is almost exactly the amount of working out you will get through the Core Program.

- Employ the Light of the Sun, page 62. With light there is no room for darkness or negative thoughts. Light is essential for life, and bringing light into your being can be a powerful tool for sustaining your body and soul during the Core Program.

The Performance Program

One of the main features of this program is going to be the addition of some appropriately timed higher intensity workouts designed to work the part of your physiology that in ancient times helped us outrun charging predators. These workouts will be the edge that bring great results in endurance sports and will also be what is necessary to fine-tune your fitness if your sport of choice is strength- or speed-oriented. Here is a partial list of activities and sports that will benefit from the Performance Program, as well as additional sports that can be maximized with this schedule:

- Competitive Running, Cycling, Swimming, and Triathlons
- Basketball
- Handball
- Track Sprinting
- High-Impact Aerobics
- High-Intensity Spin Classes
- Long Hiking and Mountain Climbing
- Downhill Skiing and High-Intensity Cross-Country Skiing
- Circuit Training

Before attempting the weekly schedule in Table 5.3, make sure that you have done a minimum of six to twelve weeks of aerobic training like we outlined in the Core Program chart. This will provide you with a strong enough base of fitness to be able to tackle the higher intensity sessions that elevate your heart rate above the MAHR.

TABLE 5.3: PERFORMANCE PROGRAM

Day	Activity	Workout Time
Monday	4 mile run, walk, or time equivalent of cycling, swimming, or other aerobic exercise.	45 minutes
	Strength Training: 2 sets of 15 reps on each exercise (see page 128).	45 minutes
Tuesday	10 minute warm-up, 40 minute cardio equipment, 10 minute cool-down.	60 minutes
Wednesday	Speed day. 10 minutes warm-up. 15–20 minutes of aerobic sport (run, swim, bike, cross-country ski, etc.) with your heart rate elevated above the aerobic maximum. This can be done continuously or broken up into interval segments in length of 1–5 minutes. Go easy between each interval for half the amount of time of that interval. (So if you do three intervals of 5 minutes of high-intensity exercise, lower the intensity for 2.5 minutes between each.) 10 minute cool-down.	50 minutes
Thursday	3 mile or 40 minute time equivalent recovery workout in the aerobic sport of your choice.	40 minutes

TABLE 5.3: PERFORMANCE PROGRAM *(continued)*

Day	Activity	Workout Time
Friday	10 minute warm-up, 30 minute cardio equipment, 5 minute cool-down. Strength Training: 2 sets of 15 reps on each exercise from the Life Strength Program (see page 128).	45 minutes 45 minutes
Saturday	Extended trail run of 6–8 miles, or equivalent amount of time in other outdoor aerobic sports (walking, mountain biking, hiking, cross-country skiing, etc.)	75–105 minutes
Sunday	Speed day. This session should be similar to what you did on Wednesday. However, mix up the length of your intervals. If you did longer ones on Wednesday, do shorter ones today, and vise versa. Note: instead of the intervals you can replace this session with an actual race or sporting event.	45 minutes

Adding in higher intensity workouts can give you huge benefits in a lot of areas of health if done correctly. High-intensity workouts promote the release of a very powerful hormone in your body called human growth hormone (HGH), which helps you build new muscle. HGH is elevated when we are infants, and then again in our teen years. These are the two times in life when a person naturally becomes significantly stronger. You can stimulate the release of this hormone at any age in large amounts if you do a hard workout—workouts that elevate your target heart rate—and by doing strength training.

Watch Out for Overtraining

While a lack of motivation or boredom can be dangerous to a fitness regimen, being overly enthusiastic about your program has its own share of pitfalls that can eventually impede your success. Overdoing intense exercise can lead to depression, short-temperedness, fatigue, muscle wasting, and a reduction in memory. Overtraining can also increase LDL (bad) cholesterol and triglyceride levels in the blood, which ultimately reduces the health of your heart and cardiovascular system.

To ensure that you don't overtrain past the point of peak fitness, be sure you fit these criteria while engaging in high-intensity workouts:

- Your sleep patterns are regular.
- You wake up feeling rested.
- You do not have lingering or abnormal muscle soreness from your anaerobic workouts.
- Your mood is good and generally stable.
- You have a normal amount of hunger—enough that you eat regular meals, but not so much that you are always hungry.
- Your workouts are consistent and it is usually easy for you to find the motivation to do them.
- You have not been sick or injured in the past two weeks.
- You have done at least two months of regular aerobic heart rate exercise prior to this regimen.

If you don't meet at least six of these eight standards, you have hit a plateau, and the only way to continue to improve fitness and health is to go back to doing strictly aerobic workouts for three to twelve weeks like you did in the Core Program. This range is wide because it will be age-dependent. Young people are more suited to absorbing the benefits from high heart rate exercise over longer periods of time than older people. This is the natural rhythm of our bodies. Young people (roughly twenty-five years and under) often get fitness gains for twelve to sixteen weeks with anaerobic workouts (high-intensity workouts) done a couple of days each week. Older people (roughly fifty-five years of age and older) can reach the maximum benefit from this kind of workout in as little as three to four weeks. Both groups will start to see deterioration in health and fitness once they reach their maximum absorbable benefit from intense levels of exercise if they continue.

Older people see improvements in fitness for long periods of time doing just aerobic workouts, while the younger people reach their maximum benefit point in a much shorter period of time.

Fit Soul Practices for the Performance Program

As with any of the Fit Soul exercises, if there are some that you find especially helpful, by all means use them to make sure your body and soul are in sync and balanced. Here are a few reminders and exercises that we find quite helpful for the periods in your training when you undertake the higher intensity workouts:

- Live What You Ask For, page 103. This is something to always remember when a fast and often painful workout is looming and resistance is creeping in. If your goal requires a high-end performance in a race or event, remember to live what you asked for. Every great performance requires this.
- Find Strength in the Nerika, page 65. Practice placing your attention in the middle of this visionary link, the doorway to your heart. See the deer person in the middle of this circle and use the peace that is in there to quiet and center your mind and thoughts. This is what separates good from great in the critical moments of competition.
- Silence the Mind, page 40. No amount of thought or mental noise can replace the benefits of your workouts, and if the internal chatter is not helping you accomplish that goal, this exercise can be used to align body, mind, and soul to work toward the same end. This can help to complete training and be practiced daily so that it becomes second nature, and a strength to draw upon during competition.

Be Smart about Recovery

No workout will do you any good if you cannot recover from it. Each time you walk, jog, lift a weight, or just move your body, there is a small amount of energy that is used and a very small amount of muscle damage that can happen. The meals we eat replace the energy stores. And then at night that glorious elixir of health called sleep is when muscle is repaired, which actually makes you stronger than you were before exercising. For most forms of exercise, one night's sleep will do the trick. But for more intense training, two or more nights of restful sleep will be required to fully repair and recover. The Huichols add a little extra recovery insurance into their lives with the world-famous siesta. The takeaway message here is that perhaps one of the most important elements to your Fit Body training is getting enough sleep to actually activate its benefits. If you need to incorporate naps into your life as you get more active, by all means do so if possible. Don't take the need or urge to sleep for granted.

Missing Workouts

In any training program there will be interruptions that prevent a workout from happening and others that need to get cut short to fit a tight life schedule. Know that this is normal. Life is unpredictable and does not necessarily follow your ideal training plan. If you find yourself pinched for time, here are some of the minimums that will significantly slow the fitness slide for quite a long period of time.

Metabolic Rate: As little as twenty minutes a day of elevating your heart rate up into your aerobic training range will keep all of your fat-burning physiology ignited. So if you're tight on time, try to fit in a short twenty-minute workout to keep the metabolic fires burning up the fat.

Strength: One set of twelve repetitions twice a week will maintain your current muscular fitness at a relatively high level, even if the goal was two sets of fifteen.

Complete Rest: After two days of complete inactivity, fitness starts to fall off gradually. So if you miss two days, try to get a workout in on the third day to stall the slide in fitness level. If this is still not possible, take heart. The drop-off is relatively small up until two weeks of no exercise. This is not an endorsement to only work out once every two weeks, but it can serve as a ray of hope that even missing a week or two of exercise will not mean starting again at the beginning.

Working with All Three Programs

You can use each of the three Fit Body Conditioning Programs throughout the year depending on your goals. If you are drawn to short burst sports (basketball, skiing, etc.) you might find that the Adaptation Program works perfectly year round as a guide for daily workout amounts, but with the addition of weekly of speed sessions found in the Performance schedule. If your base of fitness is good, you might use training volumes that are closer to the Performance Program most of the year; if you do this, be sure to only add in the speed element periodically. These are just two examples of how several of the programs can be mixed together to accomplish the Fit Body goals you are after. And as always, any of the Fit Soul exercises will benefit each of the Fit Body schedules.

Making the jump from one program to the next can be accomplished by gradually upping the total workout time over several months once you feel the need to be challenged at a higher level. Here is how you can increase your workout length, using the long workout as an example. This shows how you can make this progression in workout length over the span of nine weeks:

> Week 1: 30 minutes
> Week 2: 35 minutes
> Week 3: 40 minutes
> Week 4: 35 minutes
> Week 5: 45 minutes
> Week 6: 50 minutes
> Week 7: 45 minutes
> Week 8: 55 minutes
> Week 9: 60 minutes

This provides your body with added time for two weeks, then gives it a relative rest in the third, making longer workouts something that you work up to safely.

Achieving this in your own life can be a natural extension of the programs you already have without it having a significant time impact on your day. You may be able to add in the extra workout time after work, before returning home. It might be found at lunch, or in a workout co-op of parents with children who trade off child care duties so others can take time to exercise. Creativity coupled with desire will bring you what you need to work out.

It's the Sum of All Efforts That Matters

With the workouts in this chapter, you now have new tools to take yourself to the next level of Fit Soul, Fit Body. Use the heart rate monitor to work out in the correct training zone for increasing the base of fitness needed in all sports, to release the feel-good hormone DHEA, and to correct any overtraining imbalances that may have occurred in the past from too much high-intensity training. Add in strength training to help kick up metabolism, to add lean muscle to maintain your physiological age for years to come, and to prevent injury.

Working through the various fitness levels and adding in higher intensity workouts can be a part of that process. But going to the next level is not always about doing something new or adding in additional practices. It can be as simple as staying the course you are already on.

Use the exercises for the soul to lock in a positive attitude, to create enthusiasm for the work you have ahead, and to find gratitude for the exercise you've done already. Feel connected to your goals and your dreams, and use the power of the natural world to unite the efforts of body and soul.

We have already emphasized the value of repetition and change over time. We bring it up here again as a reminder that your next level of Fit Soul, Fit Body, of having a healthy body and a soul filled with good energy, is created with every step that you take, both the big ones and the smaller ones. You might not have the time every day for an hour-long workout or be able to devote the energy to go really deep into the exercise to connect with the light each day.

If this happens, do as much as you can. Twenty minutes of walking to and from the office is a positive step. Even thinking about the light makes a connection to it, no matter where you are when it crosses your mind. It's the sum of your efforts over time that will take you onward. It's the total of all the steps, the big ones and the small ones, that brings you health and wholeness. ✿

Huichol Prayer or Affirmation for Going On

Mother Earth, Father Sun, I give thanks that I am alive to call out to you. Give my body and my soul the desire and energy I need to go on. Embrace my being with love and light so that I can take the next steps in my journey. ✿

Chapter Six
Optimum Diet Choices
for Optimum Wellness

Eating is not optional, but the choices we have today abound. Food becomes medicine for the body and soul when wisely selected.

If there's one advantage a highly trained athlete can have over most people who lead more sedentary lives, it's being exceptionally attuned to what the body needs nutritionally. When you're training and competing at such a high level of intensity, you depend on your food and water intake to sustain your energy levels, fuel your hard-working muscles, and help you recover quickly. You can really feel the effects of what you put into your body during an endurance event, such as a blast of carbohydrates that pleases the hungry muscles and sends a rush of euphoria ("Thank you!") to your brain. But certainly more important than what you eat during a competition is refining how you eat day to day, something that becomes easier the more we make good choices in eating.

In training for my first Ironman, one of my toughest eating habits to change was giving up chocolate chip cookies. I loved them, and I could down a half dozen without flinching. I would stop by a local cookie store after my long workouts and buy five or six delicious cookies, telling myself they would last five or six days, until my next long workout. Well, you can probably guess what happened. By the time I got home there would only be one or two left.

So to avoid further temptation, I would finish those off—certainly not a good habit for someone trying to win an Ironman.

Finally it was time. I quit cookies cold turkey. Not one cookie was going to cross my lips until after the Ironman—almost six months down the road. From that moment forward, the most amazing thing happened! Everywhere I went I suddenly noticed chocolate chip cookies for sale: at the gas station, on the counter at the office supply store, at the airport, grocery store, everywhere. It was like the universe had gone mad. Or maybe I was just being tested to see if I was going to stick with my goal and live what I had committed to.

It took about six weeks, but finally I stopped seeing all those cookies for sale and my ability to fine-tune my diet with healthier choices became what I was drawn to. I went on to win my first Ironman Championship that year. I won't attribute the victory to giving up one of my toughest poor food choices, but it certainly played in my favor at the end of the day.

Functional Food, As Told by Brant

Fostering an awareness of food was also something I experienced. I developed this awareness during my time in Mexico. Don José always told me during my apprenticeship that we must remember that food's main job is to nourish the body, to give the body strength so we can carry on our daily functions in life. I remember when I was first with the Huichols one of the hardest parts about being there was the food. I was used to eating in a very different way. The Huichols eat primarily to nourish themselves. Sure they have a good time when they eat, but the food is often the same: beans and tortillas, tortillas and beans, beans and tortillas . . . and some hot sauce.

But I saw over time how this very simple diet, which provided valuable protein, brought a certain balance to my own body. Of course, we don't eat just beans and tortillas in our world here, but we can remember the message about nourishment. While indulging in rich foods is enjoyable some of the time, on a daily basis we need to ensure that we are providing the nutrient enrichment our bodies need to be healthy. And our bodies need proteins of differing sorts, which are the same proteins needed by indigenous people around the world, who know they feel strong when they eat these foods.

When I was back in America after being with the Huichols, I had to consciously work at maintaining my newfound relationship with food. I had a good time growing food in the village. It was a big part of my identity to help in the fields, to be a part of the whole process. The Huichols adoringly admire their corn and beans as they grow. The corn looks like a person, they say, with the corn silk as hair and the ears of corn as arms and legs. It's beautiful to look at. It's beautiful to think about. And then, of course, it's beautiful to eat.

In America I was forced to change my relationship with the food because I didn't (and don't) grow my own food here. I had to stay connected to that whole life process without being directly involved with it. This happened by simply doing what we emphasize in this chapter, which is to be thankful for the food. With the abundance of food in the markets, it was easy to forget to do. You'll recall my story earlier how I eventually gained fifty pounds once I started spending more time back in the U.S., and how Mark helped me work my way back to my normal weight. That reinforced the need to constantly stay aware and connected to food's functionality, as well as its sacredness.

A Universal Act

Eating is not optional, regardless of your culture, religion, body type, or fitness level. There are those who don't exercise, and others who consider a spiritual path unnecessary. But no one would put eating in the "I could live with or without it" category. Whether your home is a cave on a remote hillside or a penthouse in uptown Manhattan, we all eat.

And do we eat! Americans have soared to the top of the obesity charts worldwide. Some races are not good to win, and this is one of them. Even for those who exercise consistently, healthy eating has become a controversial mystery hidden behind fad diets, popular works of science that are regularly disproved, and a simple lack of connection to food as medicine for both body and soul.

We want to bring you back to a simple way of eating that follows our ancient genetics. This way of eating was required by our ancestors to survive thousands of years ago, and the nourishment it provides is behind every chemical reaction in our bodies. There has been no significant evolutionary adaptation that enables us to flourish on fast food or daily caloric intakes that would have fed a small village in ancient times. Relying on more traditional ways of eating can help us achieve good health more efficiently and more long-term.

The goal of eating for Fit Soul, Fit Body is to maximize the balance that food is capable of bringing you. We will help you create an eating plan that enables you to consistently make healthy choices about the types of food you eat and the correct amount for your body. You will be able to manage your weight, fuel your exercise program, and feel vibrant and healthy.

The core of this eating program involves four simple steps:

1. **Step One**: Determine Your Fit Body Eating Plan Level

2. **Step Two**: Identify Your Eating Plan Ratios

3. **Step Three**: Set Your Total Calorie Intake

4. **Step Four**: Get Portions Under Control

We're going to be walking you through each of these steps in the latter part of this chapter. As with exercise, one size does not fit all, so we will give you three different eating plan levels based on your current level of health and fitness. These levels will be used to help you determine how to approach each aspect of the eating plan. The correct balance of food group ratios, caloric intake, and portion size can make meals satisfying and help regulate weight and build muscle. It gives you clear skin, and speeds the recovery and natural buildup process after working out. It balances your hormones and blood sugar, enhances the fat profile in your blood, and will help you live a longer, healthier life with a mind that works well to the end.

With this eating plan, you can avoid the common symptoms of unbalanced eating: mood swings that can occur from eating refined carbohydrates and excessive calories, a taxed hormonal system that is created from a lack of healthy fats, and uncontrollable cravings for food—all of which can be corrected with the proper intake of protein, the hero of appetite moderators.

KEY #9:

INVITE YOUR INNER CAVE MAN TO THE TABLE

The health and weight crisis going on today, with soaring diobesity rates (the new term to describe the rise in type-2 diabetes, which is mostly caused by being overweight), boils down to the problem of primitive genetics versus modern eating. Not that our bodies are "primitive" by any means, but we are not built to withstand the rapid changes that have occurred in our food-manufacturing society.

Genetically, our bodies were set up for survival in a world where finding food was nothing like hopping in the car and driving to the convenience store at the corner. Through the millennia, the human body has not come up with a way to utilize the massive amounts and large variety of foodstuff that most of us have available just five minutes from our homes. Back when humans had to hunt and gather rather than buy their food, each season provided a handful of food items, and the amounts our ancestors could find went from surplus to shortage throughout the year. Yet we are here, so our genetics makes us experts at surviving with both food excess and food scarcity. Unfortunately for many today, we only live with the excess!

In the time of our ancestors, as today, abundant supplies of food often came in the autumn, just before the long, cold months of winter, mostly in the form of fruits, legumes, and grains that were finally ripe after a long spring and summer. For our predecessors, this season change signaled to their bodies that it was time to store up, just like bears do before hibernation. When their bodies encountered this abundance, especially of sugars, their fat-burning systems shut down, which, from the perspective of survival, makes perfect sense. If they had lots of grains and fruits to load up on just before the lean months of winter, they didn't want to keep burning their fat reserves, but rather build them up. Why eat all that food if no fat was stored?

During the winter, when only modest amounts of wildlife that could be caught and root vegetables that had been stored away were available, the opposite forces of body chemistry caused stored fat to be burned. Eating mostly protein and very little carbohydrates causes a human to utilize the hibernation layer of fat for energy (hence the short-term success of present-day high-protein, low-carb diets).

Then, once the springtime came and food sources flourished, our ancestors had an ample supply of food. There was no longer a need to gorge and store up. Instead their bodies became leaner, and metabolic rates picked back up.

Now fast forward to the modern world, where we have access to just about every food known to man, and certainly to stuff that our ancestors never saw. Cave men and cave women did not sit around sipping on Big Gulps or munching super-sized fries. However, our bodies still react to foods based on our survival genetics. If we eat lots of carbohydrates, our bodies will think that it is time to store up for the big fast during the winter and shut down the fat-burning metabolism, which results in storing the food we eat as body fat—something that most of us do not need more of. If we eat more protein and foods that don't raise our blood sugar, however, our bodies keep burning the fat at full force because, based on our ancient genetics, our bodies think that there is not a lot of food around. When this happens, our most abundant source of stored fuel—body fat—is used.

While it may seem easy to burn body fat efficiently—just eat protein and foods with low sugar density—there are several ways to throw off the body's natural fat-burning capabilities. If we eat an excess of calories in a meal (even the good calories), our bodies get a signal that food may be scarce in the near future and that it is time to store up fuel. This turns off fat burning plain and simple. Also, if we don't eat much all day but stash it away at night, based on survival genetics, our bodies interpret this as a shortage of food and hold on to every single calorie eaten to conserve, conserve, conserve. Severely restricting calories day to day (as most diet plans prescribe) also triggers our winter survival response to low food supply, again reducing the metabolic rate to help conserve energy.

How Our Cave Man Genetics Influence Our Metabolism

- A high carbohydrate diet causes the body to store fat.
- A high protein/low carbohydrate diet stimulates fat metabolism (although not necessarily a higher metabolic rate).
- High calorie intake stores body fat.
- Restricted calorie intake stores body fat.
- A huge variety in foods stimulates appetite and overall intake.
- A moderate variety of foods in modest portion sizes promotes higher metabolic rate, body strengthening, and overall body balance. ✿

If, however, we eat moderate amounts of a simple variety of foods, our bodies are at ease because this is a cue that food is in good supply and there's no longer a need to go into storage mode.

Today we are used to food being in abundance and to being able to satisfy any craving. At first, it may be challenging to make a shift in the way you eat so that you can optimize your fat-burning capabilities and fuel your workouts more efficiently.

But even before we get started on the Fit Body eating plan, it is important to understand the different food groups and how each one factors into how our body will process them.

Fit Body Food Groups: Carbohydrates, Fat, and Protein

There are three basic food groups from which you will create your meals—carbohydrates, fat, and protein. Each of these food groups is essential for life, and they work together to give you the energy you need and to provide you with the basic building blocks to keep your body healthy. If you scrimp on any one of these three food groups, your health will suffer. Likewise, if you overdo any of them, the negative effects on your health will be just as detrimental. We

> ## Good-Looking Food = Good-Looking Body
>
> Studies have shown that visually appealing food (i.e., the way it's presented) is absorbed and utilized much better by the body than the same food presented in an unappealing form. If food inspires you by the way it looks (we're not talking a giant burger and fries here), it will also inspire you to have a Fit Body and a Fit Soul.

will provide you with menu suggestions that balance these food groups, and then show you how to make balanced choices yourself.

Carbohydrates: A Fit Body's Best Friend

We are all pretty familiar with the first of our three food groups: carbohydrates. They can be found in common foods like bread, pasta, and sweet desserts. They are also naturally occurring in starchy and sweet foods from nature, like potatoes and fruit. The main job of carbohydrates is to give you energy and provide your brain with the only fuel it can use to function, which is glucose. All starches and sweets are broken down into this simple sugar before they are absorbed into our bloodstream.

In addition to keeping our brain functioning properly, carbohydrates are essential for all movement, from getting up out of a chair to racing in a competition. Even during easy to moderate intensity exercise (your aerobic workouts) carbohydrates are used to spark the reaction that breaks down fats for fuel. During high-intensity efforts, carbohydrates become the dominant source of fuel.

Carbohydrates have fallen from grace recently because of the popular low-carbohydrate diets, but every single person on this planet needs carbohydrates to live a healthy life with a well-functioning body and mind. In fact, you need carbohydrates to lose weight! You should not feel guilty every time you crave something sweet or find yourself feeling satisfied when you eat bread or sugars. Your body requires carbohydrates to survive, and the trick to Fit Body eating is knowing the right amount to include in your diet. The amount of carbohydrates that you need will vary depending on your

Top Three Food Follies

There is some conventional wisdom about good eating that can get in the way of having a truly healthy diet. Don't be fooled by misinformation or diet trends. Be aware of these food follies:

Myth: Cheese is a good source of protein.

Truth: Some cheeses get a lot more of their calories from fat—especially the unhealthy, saturated kind—than protein. Most cheese gets at least 75 percent of its calories from fat. Even though low-fat mozzarella does better at 60 percent of its calories from fat, it is still more of a fat source than a healthy protein source. The one exception is cottage cheese: a one-cup serving has about as much protein as four-ounce steak. So even though it's a dairy product, that big hunk of mozzarella cheese on your plate may not take care of all your protein needs.

Myth: Salt is bad.

Truth: It is true that salt can be unhealthy if you have hypertension, but for most people, salt can actually get depleted quite easily if you are under a lot of stress or if you work out regularly. This is not a recommendation to pour it on all over your food, but if you find your body searching for salty foods and you don't have hypertension, it may not be necessary to restrain yourself from adding it to your diet.

Myth: A low-fat diet will make you leaner.

Truth: Eating fat does not make a person fat. Dietary fat is not the same thing as fat on the body. Eating more calories than you burn through your basic metabolism and exercise is what makes a person fat. In fact, studies have shown that people on low-fat diets often put on extra body fat. The reason is that they usually replace fat calories with carbohydrate calories, which get stored as fat and depress fat burning. Remember, fat helps satisfy you and keep you feeling fuller longer. Its role in satiety is why it's important to incorporate healthy fat into every meal.

level of exercise and overall health. We will address these needs in the next section on "amounts."

The Glycemic Index

Whether you eat a potato, a piece of bread, or a candy bar, your body processes it the same way. The carbohydrates get broken down to the only form that can get from your gut to your bloodstream, which is glucose. The rate that each type of carbohydrate gets to this form is going to be key for helping you select foods that support the health goals you are after. Complex carbohydrates, like the ones in sweet potatoes, whole grain breads, legumes (such as beans), and some fruits, are all absorbed into your bloodstream slowly, which is a good thing for maintaining the body and mind balance we are after. The slower a carbohydrate gets into your blood and on its way to the cells of your body, the better.

A food's effect on the blood sugar level can be measured by the glycemic index (GI), a way to compare how the carbohydrates in various foods will affect blood sugar. Complex carbohydrates like the ones mentioned above, which release their sugar slowly, have relatively low glycemic index values (55 or less). Foods from the low and moderate glycemic categories (ones that will not cause your blood sugar to skyrocket) should make up the bulk of the carbs that you eat.

If the carbohydrates in a food break down and enter the blood stream quickly, it means that the food has a high glycemic index (70 or higher), which means that eating even a moderate amount of this food will cause a big rise in blood sugar, forcing the body to release enough insulin to bring blood sugar down (a good thing) but also enough to shut down fat burning (not a good thing). Processed foods like white sugar and corn syrup are the two most common high-glycemic foods in the modern world. Other sources of high-glycemic foods are fruit juices (even though fruit in its original form is okay) and some refined grain products like white bread. High-glycemic foods will signal your body to turn off fat burning because your body interprets the abundance of glucose in the blood to mean that it should store up fat for the upcoming winter.

If you happen to indulge in one of these carbohydrates, often called *simple carbohydrates*, the body will do its best to get your blood sugar back in balance by releasing insulin. Insulin's main job is to take extra sugar out of the blood by converting some of it into glycogen to be stored in the muscles and liver (which is good for recovery after a workout) and into fat, which will be stored in all the places on the body that most people would rather not have extra padding. This carbohydrate storage process is one reason a person can eat a very low-fat diet yet still end up having too much body fat.

Insulin turns off fat burning and shuts off the production of another key hormone that regulates blood sugar called *glucagon* (which is different from glycogen). Glucagon releases stored sugar back into the blood stream for energy and is responsible for turning on fat burning.

But when insulin is present, levels of glucagon drop in the bloodstream and fat burning is turned off. If you eat a high-carbohydrate diet regularly, you will effectively keep fat burning suppressed and make it almost impossible to lose any excess body fat, no matter how much you work out.

Table 6.1 illustrates the differences in the glycemic index of some common foods. Low-glycemic foods have a value of 55 or less and release sugar into the blood stream very slowly. Moderate-glycemic foods have values of 56–69 and release their sugar into the blood at a moderate rate. High-glycemic foods have values of 70 or greater and release sugar into the blood stream very quickly.

Change Food Chemistry in Combination

Just because a food has a high glycemic number doesn't mean it should be off-limits. You can change the entire chemistry of a meal by eating the right combination of foods. If you consume a high-glycemic food, say white bread, with a low-glycemic food, such as hummus (made up of chickpeas), what would otherwise be a quickly digested food suddenly gets slowed down in your system by the hummus. Similarly, strawberry jam (a high-glycemic food) on top of whole-grain bread won't get digested as fast, since the fiber in the bread acts like a speed bump. Which means if you want to go for

TABLE 6.1: GLYCEMIC INDEX OF COMMON FOODS

Low-Glycemic Foods (55 or less)			
Grains, Legumes, Starches	**Fruits and Vegetables**	**Dairy and Meat**	**Sweeteners and High-Glycemic Foods**
Soybeans: 20	Avocado: 0	Salmon: 0	Fructose: 22
Lentils: 29	Almonds: 0	Beef: 0	Honey: 55
Black beans: 30	Cherries: 22	Eggs: 0	Jam apricot full fruit: 55
Chickpeas: 33	Grapefruit: 25	Skim milk: 32	
Yams: 37	Apples: 38	Yogurt (fruit flavored): 33	
Pinto beans: 39	Strawberries: 40	Ice cream (low fat): 50	
Brown rice: 50	Peaches: 42	Yogurt (plain): 14	
Whole-grain bread: 51	Oranges: 44		
Pasta: 52	Grapes (green): 46	All cheeses are low-glycemic, as are milk products without added sugar.	
	Bananas: 52		

Moderate-Glycemic Foods (56–69)			
Grains, Legumes, Starches	**Fruits and Vegetables**	**Dairy and Meat**	**High-Glycemic Foods**
Basmati rice: 58	Apricots: 57		Snickers bar: 68
Pita bread: 57	Mango: 56		
Sweet potatoes: 61	Grapes (black): 59		
	Papaya: 59		
	Cantaloupe: 65		
	Corn: 56		

High-Glycemic Foods (70 and above)			
Grains, Legumes, Starches	**Fruits and Vegetables**	**Dairy and Meat**	**High-Glycemic Foods**
White bread: 70	Watermelon: 72		Rice cakes: 80
Pretzel: 83	Dates: 103		Corn Flakes: 84
Potato, baked: 85			Total Cereal: 76
Rice, Calrose: 81			
Baguette: 95			

a food high on the index, just couple it with another that's lower on the GI scale and you help minimize huge insulin swings.

Think Fiber

Developing a Fit Body is easiest when you prevent highs and lows in blood sugar from occurring by eating carbohydrates that are absorbed slowly (low-glycemic carbs). Low-glycemic carbs always have their naturally occurring fiber still intact. The more fiber a food contains, the slower it will be absorbed into your bloodstream, and the lower its glycemic score. For example, Table 6.1 illustrates that whole-grain bread, which does not include highly processed flours, has a glycemic index of 51, while a baguette, which is made of refined white flour, has a glycemic index of 95!

Men under fifty need to get at least 38 grams of fiber a day, and women under fifty need at least 25 grams. Men over fifty need only 30 grams, while women need 21 grams. Some studies suggest that consuming an extra 14 grams of fiber per day may cause the body to absorb 10 percent fewer calories. To put it simply, don't worry about eating too much fiber—it's all good for you. Whole foods make these targets easy to reach compared with process equivalents. Whole-wheat products have about 11 grams of fiber per cup, while white flour only has 3 grams per cup. Apples (consumed with their skins on) have 4 grams, while clear apple juice has virtually no fiber. The message here is that eating whole foods makes it easy to get the fiber our bodies were meant to consume. Great sources of carbohydrates that have fiber are all whole grains and legumes, including oats, beans, and corn.

In all three of the Fit Body eating plans, we will make recommendations for carbohydrate consumption based on high-fiber whole foods.

TABLE 6.2: FIBER CONTENT OF COMMON FOODS

Food	Portion Size	Grams of Fiber
Apple	1 medium	4
Pinto beans	1/2 cup dry	18.8
Black beans	1 cup cooked	19.4
Rice, white	1/2 cup dry	2
Rice, brown	1/2 cup dry	5.5
Spinach	1/2 cup cooked	7
Strawberries	1 cup	3
Yams	1 medium	6.8
Whole-wheat bread	2 slices	6
Broccoli, cooked	3/4 cup	7
Blackberries, no sugar added	1/2 cup	4.4
Lentils, brown, cooked	2/3 cup	6.4
Lentils, red, cooked	1 cup	6.4
Peas, cooked	1 cup	13.4
Cooked greens (collards, chard, dandelion)	1/2 cup	4
Figs, dried	3	10.5
Corn, cooked	1/2 cup	5
Chickpeas, cooked	1 cup	12

Fat: A Fit Body's Highest (and Heaviest) Form of Energy

Fats are absolutely essential for your existence and for sustaining a healthy body. They are one of the core necessities for maintaining healthy skin, hair, cell membranes, and just about every hormone in the body. We need fat for insulation, protection, energy, and even to think. That's right: about two-thirds of the brain is composed of fat, and the protective sheath that covers communicating neurons is 70 percent fat.

Fats come in different forms, just like carbohydrates. There are three basic types that nature has provided us with—saturated fat, monounsaturated fat, and omega-6 and omega-3 oils—and we need them all for different reasons.

Saturated Fat

Contrary to popular wisdom, a saturated fat–free diet would be detrimental to your health. Saturated fat, which mostly comes from animal and dairy products, is one of the essential compounds that a person's body needs to recover from workouts and from the daily damage that occurs naturally inside our bodies just from moving around. Saturated fat causes inflammation, which tells our bodies where damage has occurred and a repair needs to take place. Without saturated fats we would gradually deteriorate, simply because the REPAIR HERE signs would be missing inside our bodies.

Too much inflammation, however, can override its essential function in maintaining a Fit Body and cause chronic joint pain. A diet high in saturated fat can also lead to high blood pressure, heart disease, and slowing of the fat-burning system. When saturated fat builds up in the body, it can reduce the flow of the blood by constricting the blood vessels. This ends up making it more difficult to deliver oxygen to tissues and muscles, which in turn slows down your metabolism.

Few people have difficulty getting enough saturated fats in their diets, and most eat far too much. To support your Fit Body program, hold saturated fat intake to a maximum of 15 to 25 grams per day. This is how the daily recommendation measures up in food:

One ounce of cheddar cheese contains 6 grams of saturated fat

One tablespoon of butter contains 7 grams of saturated fat

A four-ounce steak contains 7 grams of saturated fat

Monounsaturated Fats

Cultures that have a diet high in monounsaturated fats are some of the healthiest in the world, regardless of their level of physical activity. A classic example of this is people who eat a Mediterranean Diet, which has olive oil as one of its staples. They have a very low rate of heart disease when compared to people who have a low intake of this special form of oil. This is not a recommendation to just sit around not exercising and just eat monounsaturated oils, but it is certainly an endorsement for their health benefits.

The champagne of all monounsaturated oils is olive oil. It is known as omega-9 oil and has some very significant positives for a person's health. It has been shown to reduce the risk of heart disease and is linked to longevity of those who eat some of it on a regular basis. It is stable inside the body and won't get converted to saturated fat like omega-6 oils can. It also stimulates fat burning and improved circulation. Extra virgin cold pressed olive oil is also high in antioxidants, which can guard against cancer and the cellular damage that can lead to cardiovascular disease.

Olive oil is the preferred choice for salad dressings and some cooking, and is much better for you than other vegetable oils, such as corn and canola oil (see the next section).

Omega-3 and Omega-6 Fatty Acids

Omega-3 and omega-6 fatty acids, which are found in the oils of many foods, reduce inflammation, which is important once damaged tissue has been repaired. The omega oils are vasodilators, which means they increase blood flow, thereby increasing the rate of oxygen delivery to the muscles. This increases fat metabolism both during exercise and also when we are just sitting quietly. Omega-3 oils come from beans, walnuts, and cold-water fish, like salmon. Omega-6 oils are extracted from vegetable and nut sources such as rapeseed (canola oil), sunflower seeds, and corn.

There is one word of caution, however, about consuming excessive amounts of omega-6 oils (commonly called polyunsaturated oils): They can be converted into saturated fat in the body if a person is under stress. Because of this, it is better to forgo many vegetable oils in favor of a monounsaturated oil for your salad dressing, such as olive oil.

The general daily requirement for omega-3 and omega-6 oils is to get roughly 2 percent of your total daily caloric intake from both of these oils. So someone eating 2,000 calories per day would need roughly 2 grams each of these two oils per day. However, some nutrition experts believe that this recommendation is not high enough and would suggest instead that people consume at least 4 percent of their total calories from these oils, or approximately 4 grams each of omega-3 and omega-6 fats daily.

Most people consume a ratio of these fats that is severely out of balance. Evidence is showing that eating these two forms of fat in a

1:1 ratio is good, and a 2:1 ratio is optimal. However, the average ratio of omega-3s to omega-6s in America is actually closer to 1:20. It is very important to balance these two oils, and the easiest way is to cut back on omega-6 sources, like canola and safflower oil, and to increase one's intake of the five best food sources of omega-3 oils, which are salmon, beans, flax seeds, walnuts, and pumpkin seeds. Here are the amounts in each of these foods:

TABLE 6.3: OMEGA-3 AND OMEGA-6 CONTENT OF COMMON FOODS

Source of Fat	Serving Size	Grams (g) of Fat
Walnuts	1/4 cup	omega-3: 2 g; omega-6: 10 g
Pumpkin seeds	4 ounces	omega-3: 7–10 g; omega-6: 20 g
Flax seeds	2 tablespoons	omega-3: 3.5 g; omega-6: 1 g
Almonds	3.5 ounces	omega-3: trace amounts; omega-6: 10 g
Salmon	6 ounces	omega-3: 3 g; omega-6: 1 g
Corn oil	10 grams	omega-6: 5 g
Flax oil	1 tablespoon	omega-3: 6.6 g; omega-6: 11 g
Butter	10 grams	omega-3: .18 g; omega-6: .12 g
Beans	1 cup	omega-3: 1 g

The World's Worst Fat: Trans Fat

Trans fat, often called "partially hydrogenated" fat, does not exist in nature. You won't find it in meat or in a plant. Yet it is in just about every processed food in the market. The idea behind trans fat is not all that bad: It is made from normally healthy oils, like canola oil, that are naturally liquid at room temperature, then its structure is changed in a process called hydrogenation. This makes it solid at room temperature. This process was developed to make oils look like butter and also to turn them into a form that works as a preservative for packaged crackers, cookies, and just about any other processed food.

So what's the catch? Partially hydrogenated fats do just about everything bad for your cardiovascular system that you can think of. They raise LDL levels (the bad cholesterol in your blood), they lower

Stock Up on Spices, Cut Back on Fat

One way to make your meals satisfying without adding extra saturated fat or omega-6 oils is by using spices. Unlike most sauces, which can be laden with fat or sugar, spices can keep the overall calorie count down and help you regulate the ratio of fats and oils in your diet. Here are a few ingredients to keep in your cupboard to spice up any snack or meal.

- Mined salt (as opposed to sea salt). Mined salt comes from ancient beds that are free of the residues that a lot of other salts have on them. If you can't find any, make sure your sea salt is free of any aluminum. The aluminum may keep your salt from caking, but keep in mind that aluminum has been linked to an increased risk of Alzheimer's disease.
- Onion powder
- Garlic powder
- Curry powder
- Soy sauce
- Cayenne and black pepper
- Salsa
- Fresh parmesan cheese (not yet grated)
- Olives and olive oil
- Walnuts

With these ingredients around the house, you can add flavor and texture to everything from tofu and soups to salads and entrees.

HDL (the good cholesterol in your blood), and they raise triglyceride levels (an indicator of a pending heart attack). Making matters worse, these fats hang around in your system for a very long time because your body doesn't have the enzymes needed to metabolize them efficiently. Increasing your total trans fat intake by as little as 5 percent leads to a 95 percent increase in your chance of having cardiovascular disease.

You have to read food labels carefully to keep from eating trans fats. Labels that claim "low fat," "low cholesterol," or "no saturated fats" do not mean there are no partially hydrogenated fats in the product. If the product has these fats included in the ingredient list (partially hydrogenated fat or trans fat) you'll want to politely put the product back on the shelf and run for the nearest healthy alternative. Fortunately, healthier options are becoming more readily available, with many stores now promoting the fact that they do not carry any products with partially hydrogenated fats. In addition, product labeling regulations are changing and soon all packaged and processed foods will be required to list how much (if any) partially hydrogenated fats are in them. Remember, if it's not found in nature, don't eat it.

Protein: A Tool in the Fit Body's Repair and Maintenance Shop

Protein has many important functions in the body, such as stabilizing blood sugar and enhancing concentration by stimulating the brain. Protein is also essential for recovery from exercise. Each workout you do does a small amount of damage to your muscles. Then, when you sleep, your body goes to work to repair that damage, using the protein from your meals. It is this repair work that lays down new muscle, making you stronger and increasing your metabolic rate, which in turn burns more body fat even when you are relaxing after a good workout.

Not all foods with protein provide the full protein spectrum needed for complete health. To do its job for repair, a protein has to be considered complete, which is a fancy way of saying that it has all the various amino acid building blocks your body will need to synthesize new protein in the body. Complete protein is found in all animal and dairy products, and in a meal that combines a grain and a legume, like corn tortillas and beans, hummus and pita bread, or whole-grain bread and nut butter. An incomplete protein (eating just a grain or a legume alone) or not eating enough protein will inhibit your body's repair process and can lead to muscle wasting.

Daily Protein Requirements

The amount of protein you need each day for optimal health depends on your weight and activity level. Here are some guidelines that can help you approximate the amount you need each day to maintain the health of your muscles, based on how much you exercise and what you weigh:

If you are sedentary: Your protein needs are going to be approximately 0.5 grams per kilogram of body weight. So for a 160-pound adult doing very little exercise, he or she will need a minimum of 36 grams of protein per day. This is roughly the amount of protein in two eggs and a three-ounce serving of salmon. (Note: pounds/2.2 = kilograms; so 160 lbs./2.2 = 72 kg. And 72 kg. x .5 = 36 grams.)

If you are moderately active: Your protein needs are going to be up to 0.7 grams per kilogram of body weight. So for a 160-pound adult doing a moderate amount of exercise, he or she will need close to 50 grams of protein per day. This is roughly the amount of protein in two servings of low-fat cottage cheese or in two eggs and a five-ounce serving of salmon.

If you are quite active: Your protein needs will go up dramatically. For the same 160-pound person, if he or she is working out for roughly an hour every day, his or her protein needs will be up to 0.9 grams of protein per kilogram of body weight per day, or roughly 65 grams of protein. This protein requirement can be met with three servings of cottage cheese, or two eggs and a sixteen-ounce serving of salmon. It also translates to about four cups of beans or lentils.

The Top Ten Fit Body Food Choices

Good, quality foods that are unprocessed, have no additives, still have their natural fiber intact, and are grown organically is what our ancient genetics is set up to thrive on. Fortunately, now more than ever before, health-conscious supermarkets, such as Whole Foods and Wild Oats, are popping up everywhere, and finding healthy food is easier than ever. Even mainstream grocery chains now have organic sections in their aisles and regularly stock what used to be considered obscure health foods, such as tofu.

TABLE 6.4: AMOUNT OF PROTEIN IN COMMON FOODS

Food	Portion Size	Protein in Grams
Salmon	3 ounces	21
Lentils	1 cup	16
Yogurt, plain nonfat	8 ounces	13
Mozzarella	1 ounce	8
Tofu	4 ounces	13
Almonds	1 ounce	6
Steak	3 ounces	24
Cottage cheese	1 cup	25
Cream cheese	1 ounce	2

Here are ten high-quality foods that you can find in any large supermarket. They will do wonders for your health and make delicious additions to your diet:

1. **Water**. Yes, this is a food, one that is often overlooked. Drinking enough will help flush your body of toxins, keep your skin fresh, help you to eat less, and keep you cool when it's hot. Dress up water by adding slices of fruit, such as lemon or lime. Try sparkling water spiked with a splash of fresh orange juice or natural (no sugar added) cranberry.

2. **Real greens**. Not iceberg lettuce, but the dark, leafy vegetables like spinach, kale, collard greens, Swiss chard, arugula, and dandelion greens. These are high in folates, which are complex substances that help our bodies absorb important nutrients, aid in cellular regeneration, and prevent cellular damage. They have also been shown to help prevent many forms of cancer and Alzheimer's disease.

3. **Extra virgin cold pressed olive oil**. This is the champagne of oils. It has an excellent profile of monounsaturated and unsaturated oil in it. It is also very stable, meaning that it will always end up being converted in the body into the basic fat elements that you need. It's also proven to be good for the heart.

4. **Flaxseed oil, walnuts, beans, and coldwater fish**. These are all very high in omega-3 oils, which help prevent heart disease. Eat these foods and you will be doing just about everything you can to keep your heart healthy through diet. In the fish department, go for wild-caught whenever possible. Wild-caught coldwater fish have a higher percentage of the good omega-3 oils and less toxins than their farmed counterparts.

5. **Soy**. Adding in tofu is an excellent way to up your protein without upping your saturated fat intake. A soy burger has 10–12 grams of protein, 1/2 cup of tempeh provides a little more than 19 grams of protein, and 1/4 cup of roasted soy nuts contains 19 grams of protein.

6. **Whole grains**. They carry a lot of fiber, making them a carbohydrate source that moderates insulin release, which is a must for fat burning.

7. **Almonds**. This simple food is gaining stature recently. It has protein and good oils, is handy to have as a snack stashed away anywhere, and is high in magnesium, which is one nutrient that people who exercise a lot are often low in.

8. **Teas—green, black, oolong**. Studies show that these teas do a great job of preventing cancer and helping to keep the bloodstream running smoothly. They also come packed with antioxidants.

9. **Food with color**. Food with color has valuable folates, which we discussed in number 2. The main food colors are yellow/orange (corn, squash, oranges), red (tomatoes, bell peppers, strawberries), green (spinach, collard greens, dandelion greens), blue/purple (blueberries, eggplant), and white (onions, garlic, leeks).

10. **Dark Chocolate**. We have to give in to one bit of decadence that is acceptable! Studies are now showing that dark chocolate has some pretty amazing positive effects on health. It improves the blood profile (increases HDL, lowers

LDL and triglycerides), fights cancer, and has been shown to produce the same feelings as being in love with another person (and love, as we know, is food for the soul). It doesn't take much to get all of these health gains from dark chocolate . . . as little as one to two ounces will get you there. Just make sure you can stop at that and not eat the whole bar. The higher the percentage of pure cocoa, the better. If you don't want to eat the chocolate, you can still use it in your quest for Fit Soul, Fit Body, by taking it like the Huichols often do—simply hold the chocolate in your hand. According to Huichol cosmology, this connects a human being to the love of Mother Earth, and helps you to develop your love for the planet.

The Ten Worst Dietary Habits

The foods we have access to can bear little resemblance to what our bodies are set up to handle and process healthily. Here is our pick for the top ten foods that are best left off your personal menu:

1. **Anything high in white, refined sugar**. Most are obvious (desserts), but some are not. Look at the label on all canned foods. Most contain either sugar or some form of corn syrup or corn sweetener. Better to get the healthy alternative.

2. **Soft drinks**. This actually comes under the previous category of white refined sugar, but it deserves its own place on the list. The "healthy" sodas, such as sparkling juices, are rarely better than the "unhealthy" ones in terms of their sugar content. They are all loaded with sugar and will most likely turn off your fat burning. Over time, drinking them regularly and in excess can lead to heart disease and diabetes.

3. **Refined flour products**. Foods like white bread have just about as good a chance of causing an insulin release because of their high glycemic index values as many noticeably sugary foods. By eating these foods instead of whole-grain

products that contain naturally occurring fiber, you increase not only your blood sugar levels, but also your risk of colon cancer. Refining takes away all the natural vitamins and enzymes that occur in the grain that help our bodies utilize it properly. Over time, eating a highly refined grain diet can lead to major imbalances in a lot of your vitamin levels, which can also end up causing ill health.

4. **Anything deep fried**. Fried foods add to the risk of heart problems and the rancid oils that most fried foods are cooked in can cause cellular damage.

5. **Nonfat desserts**. If you are going to indulge, use the full-fat originals. Nonfat means high in refined sugars and carbohydrates, which increases your chances of turning a healthy fat-burning meal into a fat-burning roadblock by releasing insulin.

6. **Anything with partially hydrogenated fat or trans fat**. This includes everything from non-dairy creamer to margarine to just about every cookie and cracker in the store.

7. **Excess carbohydrates**. Even the good ones, if eaten in excess, will be stored as fat. Only about 2,000 calories can be stored in our bodies as glycogen for later use. Every carbohydrate calorie you eat after that storage bank is full will be converted to fat. And you know where that ends up . . . exactly where you don't want it!

8. **Large meals**. Even the healthiest meal in the world will cause your body to release insulin if it is excessive in size. So eating well-balanced meals is good, but make sure the portions are in line with what your body's harmony is calling for.

9. **Any food you hate to eat**. Yes, that's right. There's a reason you do not like some foods. As you tune your dial to the real needs of what your body is calling for, it will also tell you what it does *not* want. It doesn't matter how healthy a

food is; not all healthy foods are good for all people. So if you don't like it, listen to your body and eat accordingly.

10. **Excess alcohol**. Studies have shown that a little red wine (about a glass a day) can potentially improve the blood profile in a way that decreases your chance of heart disease and many forms of cancer. However, excess alcohol, among other things, can destabilize blood sugar and disrupt sleep, which compounds the ill effects of unhealthy food cravings and any body stress you might already have.

The Fit Body Eating Plan

The Fit Body Eating Plan will complement your workout at whatever fitness level you aspire to. To help ensure you eat the diet that is appropriate to your fitness level, we have devised these four steps to the Fit Body Eating Plan:

1. **Step One: Determine Your Fit Body Eating Plan Level**. Your activity level and overall body composition will help you determine which of the three Fit Body Eating Plan levels you should begin with: Beginning Balance, Body Maintenance, or Intensive. Follow the indications for your level for each of the following three steps.

2. **Step Two: Identify Your Eating Plan Ratios**. Those who work out regularly at a high intensity will require a different balance of nutrients to nourish their bodies and build muscle than those who have been more sedentary before starting the Fit Body program. Finding the right ratios of food will help support your workout plan and achieve weight loss or muscle-building goals.

3. **Step Three: Set Your Total Calorie Intake**. Your total calorie intake will be determined by your Fit Body Eating Plan level. For those attempting to lose weight, adjusting your calorie intake will help you shed unwanted pounds.

4. **Step Four: Get Portions Under Control**. Eating the correct portions of protein, fat, and carbohydrates will help you achieve nutrient balance and support your workouts.

Step One: Determine Your Fit Body Eating Plan Level

The first step is to identify where you are on the BMI chart on the next page (Table 6.6). Then compare that number to the corresponding range in Body Composition and Risk Factor Chart below (Table 6.5). After calculating your BMI, you can use it to help you find the Fit Body Eating Plan level that is right for you with Table 6.7.

TABLE 6.5: RISK OF ASSOCIATED DISEASE ACCORDING TO BMI AND WAIST SIZE

BMI	Weight Status	Risk level if waist is less than or equal to 40 inches (men) or 35 inches (women)	Risk level if waist is greater than 40 inches (men) or 35 inches (women)
18.5 or less	Underweight	N/A	N/A
18.5-24.9	Normal	N/A	N/A
25.0-29.9	Overweight	Increased	High
30.0-34.9	Obese	High	Very High
35.0-39.9	Obese	Very High	Very High
40 or greater	Extremely Obese	Extremely High	Extremely High

Beginning Balance

Those who will most benefit from this eating plan are those who are either over their healthy weight or are just starting out with a training program after a long period of being inactive, or both. If a lack of exercise is part of this picture, it is important to eat a diet that is lower in overall carbs in the beginning.

Even someone who is fairly lean may not be able to metabolize carbohydrates well. The reasons for being lean can come from positives in life—exercising, eating good foods, getting plenty of rest, and maintaining a low-stress, happy, Fit Soul lifestyle—but can also

TABLE 6.6: BODY MASS INDEX (BMI)

BMI	19	20	21	22	23	24	25	26	27	28	29	30	35	40
Height (in.)						Weight (pounds)								
58	91	96	100	105	110	115	119	124	129	134	138	143	167	191
59	94	99	104	109	114	119	124	128	133	138	143	148	173	198
60	97	102	107	112	118	123	128	133	138	143	148	153	179	204
61	100	106	111	116	122	127	132	137	143	148	153	158	185	211
62	104	109	115	120	126	131	136	142	147	153	158	164	191	218
63	107	113	118	124	130	135	141	146	152	158	163	169	197	225
64	110	116	122	128	134	140	145	151	157	163	168	174	204	232
65	114	120	126	132	138	144	150	156	162	168	174	180	210	240
66	118	124	130	136	142	148	155	161	167	173	179	186	216	247
67	121	127	134	140	146	153	159	166	172	178	185	191	223	255
68	125	131	138	144	151	158	164	171	177	184	190	197	230	262
69	128	135	142	149	155	162	169	176	182	189	196	203	236	270
70	132	139	146	153	160	167	174	181	188	195	202	207	243	278
71	136	143	150	157	165	172	179	186	193	200	208	215	250	286
72	140	147	154	162	169	177	184	191	199	206	213	221	258	294
73	144	151	159	166	174	182	189	197	204	212	219	227	265	302
74	148	155	163	171	179	186	194	202	210	218	225	233	272	311
75	152	160	168	176	184	192	200	208	216	224	232	240	279	319
76	156	164	172	180	189	197	205	213	221	230	238	246	287	328

TABLE 6.7: FIT BODY, FIT SOUL EATING PLAN ASSESSMENT

BMI	Little or No Exercise (Less than 4 days and/or less than 3 hours of total exercise per week)	Moderate Exercise (4–6 days and 6–10 hours of total exercise per week)	Intensive Exercise (6–7 days and/or 12 or more hours of total exercise per week)
18.5 or less	Maintenance	Intensive	Intensive
18.5-24.9	Maintenance	Maintenance	Intensive
25.0-29.9	Beginning	Maintenance	Intensive
30.0-34.9	Beginning	Beginning	Maintenance
35.0-39.9	Beginning	Beginning	N/A
40 or greater	Beginning	N/A	N/A

come from the negatives. These include a high-stress lifestyle, lack of sleep, starvation dieting, and loss of lean muscle mass caused by not enough exercise or from long periods of high-intensity exercise that also cause muscle wasting. In all of these cases, simply strapping on the heart rate monitor and seeing what your aerobic pace is while running will tell you if you are able to burn fats efficiently. If your pace is slower than about a twelve-minute mile, you will probably benefit greatly from this dietary plan. If you prefer to gauge your aerobic capacity by doing something other than running, then just engage in the physical activity of your choice and see if you feel winded or physically extended. If your face turns red and you feel out of breath quickly, then the Beginning Balance is for you.

Remember, one goal of how we eat is to help stimulate our body's ability to utilize fat for its main source of fuel. This will also support one of the goals of our Fit Body training, which is to build the aerobic fat-burning engine. It will also be a very important ingredient supporting one of the main goals of our Fit Soul Program, which is to bring stability to our emotional state. And one of the best ways to support that through diet is to stabilize blood sugar levels, which is a very important element of the Beginning Balance Program.

The metabolism in a person who is overweight or sedentary acts as though there is little food available and causes the body to hold on to precious body fat and to cut back on muscle building as a way to conserve energy. We want to reverse this inefficient metabolic process with the Beginning Balance Program by providing enough balanced nutrition to shift your metabolism into fat-burning mode.

Portion control and the total amount of calories consumed per day are important for those who are attempting to lose weight. Once you start working out and following the Fit Body Eating Plan, there are some important factors you need to keep in mind.

Don't Go Below 1,500 Calories per Day: It's extremely important to make sure that the daily amount you eat is no fewer than about 1,500 calories for men or 1,200 calories for women. Eating fewer calories than this tricks the body into thinking it's starving to death. Your metabolism will plummet as the body enters self-preservation mode, and the amount of calories you burn each day will also go down dramatically. By eating too little food your body will hold on to every piece of good food you put into it, and chances are that all the weight and more will come back in about a quarter of the time it took you to lose it. The lesson: keep your metabolism humming by giving your body the energy it needs to operate efficiently.

Be Mindful of Calories, Even After Exercise: Keep in mind that increasing exercise will generally increase hunger. Make sure that your food intake doesn't overtake your increase in workouts.

Trim Carbohydrate Portions First: If you're having trouble losing weight even though you're working out as much as you can, try cutting your portion size back by 10 to 15 percent for a couple of weeks and see what happens. Eating slowly and enjoying your good food will make the reduction in portion size virtually unnoticeable. If you are going to trim portion sizes, it is best to start with reducing your carbohydrates and trying to keep the protein and oil components stable. If this still does not produce a desired shift in body composition, gradually decrease the serving sizes of all three components of your food choices.

If your current BMI and fitness level put you into this Beginning Balance category, follow the guidelines given for Body Balance in the Ratio, Total Calorie Intake, and Portion Size sections below. The Adaptation Program in Chapter 5 is an ideal complement to the Body Balance eating plan.

Body Maintenance

The Body Maintenance level of the program is designed for those who are healthy and active, yet haven't reached the peak fitness levels they desire. People in this category may also struggle to lose those "last five or ten pounds." This plan will provide enough carbs to regenerate muscle after activity (the energy from carbohydrates is required to synthesize new muscle) but not so many that your body will start storing them as fat.

If your current BMI and fitness level put you into this category, follow the guidelines given for Body Maintenance in the Ratio, Calorie Intake, and Portion Sizes sections below. The Core Program in Chapter 5 is an ideal complement to the Body Maintenance eating plan.

Intensive Program

The good news for the few who exercise more than about an hour and a half a day is that they will be quite good at processing carbohydrates without big insulin responses. This is why athletes can eat all kinds of junk and still stay lean and strong looking. The reverse of this is that with a higher activity level, to stay healthy and not metabolize your lean muscle for energy, you will need to eat more calories and more carbohydrates in relation to your fat and protein.

A big factor for many people who work out at this level is staying well hydrated. Weigh yourself before and after a workout. For every pound lost, you will need to drink one and a half pounds of fluid to replace what you just sweated out. And what a treat, as water is sacred and makes our body and soul beautiful!

If your current BMI and fitness level put you into this category, follow the guidelines given for Intensive in the Ratio, Total Calorie Intake, and Portion Sizes sections below. The Performance Program in Chapter 5 is an ideal complement to the Intensive eating plan.

Step Two: Identify Your Eating Plan Ratios

Table 6.8 provides the percent of overall calories that should be consumed of carbohydrates, protein, and fats for each of the three plan levels. As you can see, the biggest shifts happen in the overall ratio of carbohydrates in each of the three plans. As we described, the Beginning Balance level will help improve carbohydrate metabolism, which in turn will aid in aerobic fitness development and can ease hormonal swings. The carb intake at the Body Maintenance level sustains an equilibrium for someone who already has generally good health and fitness, but who is not taxing their body with extreme fitness demands. The ratio of carbs in the Intensive level will help replenish depleted carb reserves that are essential to keep stocked up for working out and also for muscle regeneration that takes place during recovery from longer training bouts.

TABLE 6.8: EATING PLAN RATIOS

FBFS Eating Plan	Percent of Daily Calories from Carbohydrates, Protein, and Fat		
	Carbohydrates	Protein	Fat
Beginning Balance	40	30	30
Body Maintenance	50	25	25
Intensive	60	20	20

Step Three: Set Your Total Calorie Intake

Eating the right amount of food for your body is about the most important task facing the modern world food scene. We have super-sized our plate expectations far from the scale of what our ancestors looked for in their meals. Even in the last twenty-five years, food intake in America has increased by 30 percent. The amount of food that will support your best health and recovery is based on your weight and exercise level and can be calculated using the following table:

TABLE 6.9: TOTAL CALORIE INTAKE

Program	Calories Needed Per day
Beginning Balance	12–14 per pound of body weight
Body Maintenance	15–17 per pound of body weight
Intensive	18–24 per pound of body weight

Taking all of this into account, if you are just starting out and weigh 190 pounds, the amount of food that you will need is roughly 190 x 13 or about 2,500 calories. If you have a partner who weighs 110 pounds and is working out at a moderate level, that person's needs will be 110 x 16 or about 1,700 calories per day.

If your BMI is 30 and your partner's is 20, the ratios of carbohydrates, protein, and fats from those calories will differ as well. You will be best served by the Beginning Balance Plan, and your partner the Body Maintenance Program. Each one will look like this in terms of total amounts during a one-day period:

2,500 calories at a ratio of 40:30:30 = 250 grams carbs, 185 grams protein, and 85 grams fat

1,700 calories at a ratio of 50:25:25 = 150 grams carb, 105 grams protein, and 47 grams fat

Determining Total Calories

Each of our foods yield a specific number of calories. Carbohydrates give off four calories per gram. The same goes for protein. Fats pack a wallop, giving the body nine calories for every gram. So when comparing apples to apples on food packages, make sure to either compare total calories from each of the nutrients, or to convert the grams of each into calories so that you can have a better idea of the ratio of carbs to protein to fat that is in your grocery bag.

Step Four: Get Portions Under Control

If you were to ask us for the "secret" to weight loss, or the only weight-loss plan that works, we'd tell you to watch your portions. There have been and still continue to be diet plans marketed that say they have found the solution to why people have gained weight, and offer the road back to lean and mean. However, in the long run (meaning after any shock regime of the diet has been passed), the only eating plan that has been proven to work over time is portion size reduction. All long-term weight loss, especially that which is stable, comes about through moderating portion size. Of course, this can be enhanced by what is in those portions, but smaller portions is the bottom line on getting your body where you want it—and keeping it there.

Knowing the nutrient content of the foods you eat will help you determine the portion sizes you should eat of carbohydrates, protein, and fats. We understand that it's unrealistic to make this a complicated process, or to turn your kitchen into a lab where you measure out precise portions with scales and calculators. Instead we're going to give you a few guidelines that will help you to make good decisions about portions. You should already have an idea based on the previous charts how many calories you should be consuming each day, and the ratio of those calories that should be coming from each food group—proteins, carbohydrates, and fats. Use the chart below to help you gain an understanding about the makeup of different types of foods.

The Plate Method

One of the easiest ways to get your portions under control is to use the plate method, which is how a lot of dieticians and nutritionist teach their clients to measure out proper portions. Divide your plate into sections based on three things: 1) sources of **non-starchy vegetables**, 2) sources of **lean protein**, and 3) sources of **whole grains, starchy vegetables, fruit, and dairy**. You do this because it's simply not practical to section off a plate by food groups—fat, for example, can be found in both your protein and carbohydrate sources. Likewise, carbohydrates will be found largely in vegetables and grains. But you'll want to have a source of protein at every meal, and because it's critical to get plenty of colorful fruits and vegetables into your diet

> Note: For those who are interested in taking the more precise route, we have created a shortcut for doing the math on exact portions. That information and the related chart is posted on our Web site www.fitsoul-fitbody.com. But it's not necessary. The goal is for you to become so attuned to your body that you know what a proper size is for you, and you can build your own meals effortlessly.

TABLE 6.10: FIT BODY PORTIONS

Food	Serving Size	Calories	Protein grams	Carbohydrate grams	Fat grams
Common Protein Sources					
Meat, fish, poultry	4 ounces	229	34	0	9
Eggs	1 large	75	6.3	0.6	5
Nonfat milk	8 ounces	86	8.4	11.9	0.4
Yogurt, nonfat plain	8 ounces	110	12	16	0
Tofu, firm	1/2 cup	183	19.9	5.4	11
Beans, lentils, and other legumes	1/2 cup, cooked	117	7	21.8	0.4
Cottage cheese, low fat	1/2 cup	90	14	4	2.5
Mozzarella, part skim	1 ounce	80	8	1	5
Parmesan	1 tablespoon	25	2	0	1.5
Cheddar	1 ounce	110	7	1	9
Nuts	1 ounce	170	6	5	14
Common Carbohydrate Sources					
Bread, whole-grain	2 slices	70	3	16	1
Potato, baked with skin	1 average	119	2.5	27.4	0.1
Rice, corn, and other grains	1/2 cup, cooked	160	4	34	0
Corn	1/2 cup	80	3	20	0
Oats	1 cup, cooked	145	6	25.2	2.4
Beans, lentils, and other legumes	1/2 cup, cooked	117	7	21.8	0.4
Vegetables	1/2 cup	22	2.3	3.9	0.2
Cakes and muffins	1 piece	300	5	38	19
Pastas	2 ounces, uncooked	200	7	41	1
Berries	1/2 cup	23	0.5	5.2	0.3
Bananas	1/2 cup	104	1.2	26.4	0.5
Apples	1 average	80	0.3	21.1	0.5
Honey, maple syrup, sugar, and other sweeteners	1 ounce	110	0	28.3	0
Common Fat Sources					
Oils	1 tablespoon	120	0	0	14
Butter	1 tablespoon	100	0.1	0	11

for their vitamins, minerals, fiber, antioxidants, and other nutrients, it helps to devote a section on your plate to filling up on these.

Here's how to section off your plate and fill it up using this method:

1) Section 1: Non-starchy vegetables—fill about half of your plate with vegetables, leafy greens, spinach, broccoli, asparagus, bell peppers, cucumber, etc.

2) Section 2: Lean proteins—fill a little less than a quarter of your plate with lean proteins like meats, seafood, and poultry, or with a properly combined gain and legume. About 3 to 5 ounces is ideal, which translates to an amount the size of your palm or a deck of cards.

3) Section 3: Starches—fill about one-quarter of your plate with low-glycemic starches, fruit, or dairy products. Starchy vegetables like squash, yams, potatoes, and corn are also included in this category. Opt for whole-grain choices wherever possible.

You'll notice that this method brings the plate up to almost 100 percent. That last bit of space is where you can add healthy fats, such as a drizzle of olive oil on your greens, a sprinkle of nuts and seeds, or a wedge of avocado. This is not an exact science, so don't feel like you have to draw lines on your plate. Having a sense of an ideal portion for you body's needs is the key to achieving Fit Body goals, and that comes with practice and by tuning in to your body's inner signals of hunger and satiety at every meal.

Now you may be wondering how to combine the key formulas here: the number of calories you should be consuming per day; the ratio of carbs, protein, and fat from those allotted calories per day; and this plate method. The most straightforward way to do this is to be mindful of your ratios, and when you look at your self-designed plate, visualize the breakdown. Let's do an example.

Let's say you're in the Beginning Balance category. You should be consuming 40 percent of your calories from carbohydrates, 30 from protein, and 30 from fat. When you look at the calories on your lunch plate—a salad with lettuce, dandelion greens, raw almonds, olive oil, and tuna, plus crackers with feta on the side—you find that less than half of the total calories on the plates (40 percent) are in the greens and crackers, and more than half of the remaining calories are split evenly between the fat (olive oil; 30 percent) and proteins (tuna, almonds, and feta; 30 percent). There's lots of flexibility with which to play throughout your day. You don't have to create meals that adhere rigidly to your daily ratios of carbs, protein, and fat. The goal is to hit your target numbers by the end of the day.

Now, the next question to ask yourself is: How *big* is this salad? Again, this will depend on your calorie-intake level. If you're aiming to consume only 1,500 calories a day, then you need to keep the portion small. The more calories allotted for you, the bigger your portions can be. Simple as that.

Fill Up on Fiber and High-Quality Protein

Once trick to use when you've eaten a decent portion but still feel hungry is to add a little more protein and fibrous vegetables to your plate, rather than more carb-rich grains. You're more likely to fill up faster on protein and fiber than if you were to drop another dollop of rice or pasta onto your plate. By "high-quality protein," we mean lean sources, like those from non-fat dairy products and white meats, as opposed to red meats marbled with fat.

Intuitive Eating

The ability to get in touch with our bodies and know exactly how much fuel we need to run efficiently is in each and every one of us— guaranteed. Just think about it . . . over the course of a year most of us will eat over a million calories! How did our ancestors go from start to finish of this 365-day cycle with almost no significant change in body weight? Because our bodies will tell us what to eat for optimal health if we listen correctly. Long before tables that calculate food content, portion sizes measured to the gram, and body composition charts, people were able to maintain great health, optimum fitness, and a peaceful soul, all nourished by natural foods.

The following are two additional Fit Soul exercises to help you tap in to that intuitive common sense that many of us have lost when it comes to eating. Each one will work to help counter some of the reasons people eat, reasons that have little to do with nourishing the body but rather come from emptiness in our soul. Use these two exercises in times when you feel yourself reaching for something to fill up an emptiness that has more to do with emotions than calories.

Feeding Your Soul with Love Exercise

- Sit down on Mother Earth and visualize yourself in the middle, between earth and sky. Think about who you are as a person, and that you have love inside of your body as an inherent quality. The love you have as a human being connects you to the four directions.
- Imagine yourself breathing in love from each of the four cardinal directions—east, south, west, and north.
- Visualize the feeling or spirit of love coming through a doorway or tunnel from the east that goes directly into your soul, at your heart level. Feel this love spread like a flame throughout your body. Feel how this love feeds your soul. Fill yourself up with the spirit of love, kindness, and compassion. This all helps to make you whole or complete.
- Do the same for each of the four directions. Feel your connection to each one. You can physically face each direction or not. It is up to you. This simple exercise can help to fill any emptiness in your soul with love rather than with food, which is important in everyone's life.

Feeding Your Soul with Community Exercise

- Visualize yourself in the center of a circle surrounded by people you know, both intimately and perhaps casually. These people are all part of your community (or we might say it's your *tribe*). The circle is made up of people that you are close to, including both family and friends.
- Try to feel yourself connected to each person by energy, like the spokes in a wheel. You are in the center and are indeed connected to all people you come in contact with, and thus you feed your soul with community, friends, or loved ones.

Sample Meals

Corn, beans, salsa, and fresh fruits and vegetables would meet just about every one of our body's requirements for food, but most of us in the modern world like to have a diverse variety of tastes in our meals. Below is a suggested weekly meal plan composed of foods that will nourish your body. Each meal has a balance of our three main nutrients, and each one comes from a healthy source. The actual amount of food that you eat will be based on your daily caloric needs. Feel free to add in snacks so you're not going more than four hours without eating (ideas on this coming up). If you remember to eat something every three to four hours, you will keep your metabolism humming and your blood sugar stable, and you won't feel uncomfortably famished or stuffed.

Monday

- Breakfast: Omelet with tomato, avocado, and salsa. Toast with almond butter and fruit spread.
- Lunch: Hummus and hard crackers. Arugula with olive oil, walnuts, and grated parmesan cheese.
- Dinner: Either salmon or Cajun red beans, with basmati rice and broccoli. Tomato and mozzarella with olive oil.

Tuesday

- Breakfast: Whole grain flake mix (corn flakes, millet flakes, etc.) with sunflower and flax seeds. Yogurt, honey, and berries.
- Lunch: Salad with lettuce, dandelion greens, raw almonds, olive oil, and either tuna or beans. Crackers with feta.
- Dinner: Pasta with squash, parmesan cheese, olive oil, and either tempeh or chicken. Tomato and avocado with cracked pepper.

Wednesday

- Breakfast: High-protein pancakes with natural maple syrup. Yogurt and berries.

- Lunch: Curry tofu on crackers with grated carrots, olives, and scallions. Apple.
- Dinner: Either green lentils or chicken with parmesan cheese, sautéed spinach, and basmati rice. Yogurt with fruit spread.

Thursday

- Breakfast: Fruit and yogurt smoothie with flax seeds. Whole-grain toast with almond butter and fruit spread.
- Lunch: Lemon chickpea soup with summer squash and tomatoes over couscous. Apple.
- Dinner: Spicy sauté with either tofu or beef, tomatoes, and peanut sauce. Basmati rice. Salad with lettuce, arugula, walnuts, and olive oil. Berries and yogurt.

Friday

- Breakfast: Frittata with tomatoes, feta, and olives. Whole-grain toast with almond butter and fruit spread.
- Lunch: Corn tortillas with beans, tomatoes, avocado, salsa, and low fat cheddar.
- Dinner: Pasta with sautéed tomatoes, onions, and basil. Olive oil. Side of either seared salmon or sautéed spicy tofu.

Saturday

- Breakfast: Bagel with light cream cheese and either smoked salmon and tomato or hard crackers with feta, olives, and tomato. Yogurt with fruit spread and berries.
- Lunch: Sautéed greens and walnuts. Lentil soup with parmesan cheese and sourdough bread topped with feta.
- Dinner: Basmati rice and sautéed tomatoes and onions with either spicy daal or spicy chicken. Yogurt dill sauce.

Sunday

- Breakfast: High-protein French toast with berries and natural maple syrup. Yogurt.

- Lunch: Either sesame tuna or turmeric tempeh over Swiss chard and tomatoes with pine nuts and parmesan cheese. Hard crackers with olive spread.
- Dinner: Spicy Thai chicken or tofu with broccoli, tomatoes, and walnuts over pasta. Mandarin oranges with yogurt.

Additional Stragegies for Fit Body Eating

Healthy Eating Starts at the Store

Not all stores are created equal. While most are beginning to offer healthy choices in products, some may still tempt you with a processed food jungle. If you should find yourself in one, here's a great tip: Stick to the outer aisles of the market. This is where you usually find the good stuff. The inner aisles normally house the processed foods, so stay away from those and shop on the perimeter of the store for good health. Obviously health food stores have different criteria for shelving. The message is to just be alert no matter where you shop.

Just Say No to Speed Eating

Sometimes we approach getting through a meal like we plow through a stack of bills—the quicker the better. But eating is not a speed sport, and speed eaters are overeaters. Eating slowly gives the food time to start digesting and move out into your body as you are eating. This helps the hunger meter to hit "satisfied" with a much smaller amount of food still waiting in your stomach to be digested. It will also help you stop eating at the point where you feel satisfied as opposed to stopping when you feel full, because food's good taste is always noticed most in the beginning of a meal and slowly diminishes as our bodies start to absorb nutrients. After that point, that initial burst of great taste wanes, which is nature's way of saying "enough." We can miss that switch when we are power eating at top speed, only stopping when the tank is filled to the top, which is well beyond the level we need to sustain and nourish our bodies healthfully. There is a subtle yet important distinction in knowing when to say enough. And before the first bite, just remember with gratitude all that went into that food to get it to your plate.

Eating for a Fit Soul: Remembering Where Food Comes From

When preparing to eat a meal, try to remember the sacred journey your food has taken from seed to saucer, and give thanks for the way it will give health to your body. Corn, for example, is nourished gently with water as it germinates inside the earth. It takes in the love of Mother Earth just as we do and begins to grow. The air feeds the seed, as does the warmth and light of the sun. It takes in the four elements for months as it prepares itself for you. This is a long process, and by remembering it with all that you eat, your soul becomes aware of why you eat. It can then help you to make healthy choices for your body's nourishment because you remember the sacredness of food.

Before that first bite, give the food laid out in front of you your attention, some conscious focus. Try for at least part of the meal to leave work, worries, and the headaches of life behind and remember that what is passing between your lips will end up in your stomach and to all points beyond. When you see eating as a sacred act that is done in a conscious way, the food has a different effect on the body. The food is then more nourishing.

Turn Your Cravings into Healthy Eating

When most people get a food craving between meals, often the first image that comes to mind is something sweet. But as you learned, carbohydrates can cause blood sugar swings that give a short-term feeling of being satiated but lead to craving more later. An alternative to this is to snack on food that has a modest amount of carbohydrates but also a good amount of protein. A great way to boost the protein without having to worry about increasing your saturated fat intake is to get your complete protein through food combining, as we discussed earlier (grains plus legumes, grains plus nuts or seeds, legumes plus nuts or seeds).

Here are a couple of snack ideas based on these guidelines:

- Hummus and crackers
- Almond butter on toast with fruit-sweetened spread
- Walnuts on salad with lentils
- Tortillas and beans with avocado
- If these don't do the trick, one of the best standbys is low-fat plain yogurt that you can add your own sweetener to if desired.

Balanced Eating, Balanced Body

Good food in the right ratio of carbohydrates, proteins, and fats will balance your body. Eating the right amount of food will give you energy, help you maintain a healthy body composition, and allow you to recover effectively from exercise, no matter what level. Feeding your soul with love, stepping out of isolation and into community, and giving thanks for the sacredness of food all stimulate your body's intelligence, which whispers the right foods for you to eat for nourishment, and will allow your meals to become medicine for both body and soul. We encourage you to use the information in this chapter as your launching pad to better eating, first "walking," by using the charts, and then eventually "running," by listening to your body and what it is telling you to eat for your best health, balance, and well being. *Bon appétit!*

Chapter Seven
Discover a Life Without Limits

Being steady nurtures the soul.

Which would you rather be, the proverbial tortoise or the hare? Well, based on how the story ends, logically you'd pick the patient tortoise . . . because you know that slow and steady wins the race!

When I was racing competitively in triathlons, I often found that the steadiest athletes—the "tortoises"—always had the best performances. Race reports are littered with names of athletes who were fast in the beginning, experiencing the high of an early lead, but who crashed and burned later when they ran out of energy. The winners were often seemingly out of the picture in the first half of the race, but then crept into the standings near the end of the bicycling segment, and then passed everyone with ease late in the marathon to win.

I was the high-and-low athlete during the first half of my career. Then, fortunately, Brant's teachings opened up an entirely different perspective on strength—that there is strength in being steady. It took self-confidence to let the others get ahead in the early stages of the race, and a certain amount of humility to hold back until the time was right. But then as the others wore down, steadiness paid off. And the dividends were immeasurable!

In the last two chapters, we gave you techniques geared mostly toward achieving a physically fit body. These include doing the bulk of aerobic exercise at moderate heart rates (*slow down to get faster*), utilizing strength training, and eating a good diet attuned to your nourishment needs. Complementing this by using the Fit Soul exercises outlined in earlier chapters, we have also shown you how to clear the way for these physical transformations to be possible, such as paying attention to joy, transforming negative thoughts into positive ones, remembering gratitude, and making connections to community and to the healing power of nature.

This combination of body and soul focus can be used for a short period to bring about positive changes in health and well-being, or it can be incorporated into your lifestyle every single day you have left on this beautiful earth. Somewhere in that journey you might decide that you want to make bigger changes in your health and your personal goals. We all have comfort zones that can become easy to work within, but sometimes an inspiring thought lies well beyond those normal borders. Suddenly we may find ourselves thinking "outside the box." For instance, you might want to achieve a much higher level of performance—whether it's in a sport, at work, or on a deeper, spiritual level. There might be a vision of personal growth that you have shied away from because of not believing you could succeed in getting there.

Well, it's time! We want to give you special, additional techniques that will help propel you beyond any limits of body and soul you might have felt or experienced before. This can be a very exciting and gratifying part of your journey as you broaden your personal experience of Fit Soul, Fit Body in a natural but powerful way. We've given you a wealth of information and strategies up to this point to help develop a Fit Soul and Fit Body, including the nine main keys.

Clearly, however, there are more keys to living a happy, fit life; we chose those nine in particular because they provide a great foundation from which to build and continue to expand. Finding strength in steadiness is just one example of another key that extends naturally from that core foundation. In this chapter we'll offer additional focal points for success, including practices and exercises to help you find your own strength in steadiness.

On the surface, this may sound like it's going to be a call for more, *more*, *MORE*. More exercise, more time devoted to developing your soul, more things that have to get done before you end up where you want to be. And indeed there may be the need to up your commitment to doing the work necessary to take your life to a new place. But tapping in to a limitless life can also be as simple as replacing an old way of doing things with a new perspective on life or a more effective workout style. So before you start thinking that the suggestions are going to be unrealistic, take heart. Living a life beyond limits can be as simple as modifying your approach or perspective ever so slightly. And then the draining thought of impossibility vanishes.

With a Strong Foundation, There Are No Limits

A life beyond limits begins with a few simple thoughts or affirmations of possibility, ones that say "I can. I can take the energy of my good work and thoughts and use them to live a simple yet extraordinary life beyond any limits I may have felt before." We see the "impossible" take place over and over in the world all around us, but we often take it for granted. A leaf transforms the energy of the sun into nourishment. We eat food and transform its energy into fuel for our bodies. These simple yet profound events happening every moment of the day can be used as a model for our own ability to change.

Huichol cosmology gives us many images of transformation that can guide us as well. For example, according to their tradition, before human beings existed, Grandfather Fire walked all over the earth and sang sacred songs of creation that turned energy into matter, such as mountains, lakes, and springs. Another ancient Huichol story of transformation tells of how the sun came into being. According to this legend, the sun was once a young girl who magically transformed into a man and then was miraculously transformed into Father Sun. This is why in the Huichol tradition the sun is said to be a man with the soul of a young girl.

These two simple stories reveal the idea of creating something completely unbelievable through a mystical transformation. They are told and retold to the people of their community and become a model for each person to follow throughout life, one that does not place limits on what can be accomplished. This concept of using inspirational stories is certainly familiar in the modern world. The stories of great athletes inspire younger ones to strive for excellence. Stories of triumph over disaster inspire hope in the hearts of humanity. It's one natural way to take a thought ("I can"), an image (a seed turning into a giant tree), or a story (the sun once being a young girl) and have it inspire your own transformation, to take you to a new place beyond your personal limits.

Challenge Your Limits: Create a New Concept of Normal

We have talked about how goals can be the magnet that draws you into consistent action, to be the carrot that keeps you going day to day. But a goal can sometimes become an invisible kind of boundary or limit. It can be a target that becomes the "normal" place we are reaching for. It is often these concepts of normal that keep you from exploring new ground. But changing your perspective by redefining what can be normal for you can free you from any self-imposed limits. One way to do this is to completely interrupt your normal behavior with a favorable, but extreme, change—whether in exercise, food, or soul—for a short period of time. Then, gradually return to your former normal behavior. You will discover that what you once considered normal no longer feels empowering, and you are able to be more active or eat healthily beyond your previous limits. Here are examples of how to do this:

Be Consistent. Consistency is a close cousin to steadiness, and a theme we've mentioned previously in the book. Sometimes we have the feeling of always starting over, week after week, simply because life interrupts our plans for working on body and soul. Reset this pattern with a one-week commitment to consistency. For seven days in a row, do a workout, which can be as simple as going for a brisk stroll after dinner each night. Every day for one week take the time to stop and be aware of the sunrise or the sunset. Even if your consistency takes the form of the shortest of workouts or just a few moments outside when the sun goes down to take in the wondrous colors, that will be fine. Something is better than nothing, and more importantly, it will signal to your body and soul that consistency is possible. As much as steadiness won the race for the tortoise, so did consistency.

Be Conscious of Every Thought. Psychologists have proven that we have upward of 60,000 thoughts a day, and the vast majority of those are negative! To improve your efficiency at curbing negative thoughts that affect your soul, for three days be conscious of everything you tell yourself. If you find a negative thought comes in, immediately replace it with a positive statement. This may seem tedious, but at the end of the three-day period the frequency of incoming negatives will be significantly less than what used to be your norm.

Watch What You Eat. If you eat too many carbohydrates, cut out all sweets, pasta, and breads for three to seven days. Then slowly add more varieties of healthy carbs, the ones with all their fiber still intact, into your diet. As you gradually begin to eat carbs again, you will find that you are satisfied with a smaller amount of healthier carbohydrate foods than you were before.

Move More. To reset a workout boundary, for two weeks increase your workout time one day a week by 50 percent. This will definitely feel challenging. Then in the third week, reduce your increased workout by 25 percent. What you will experience now is that the 25 percent reduced workout feels easier than your original long workout. You have a new "normal"!

Steadiness Is Empowerment

A Huichol model you can use to live beyond normal limits is to keep focusing on the thought of staying steady. The entire Huichol culture is steady—steady in life, steady with their emotional character, steady with how they embark on any task. This is a focus that can help you navigate any barriers, borders, or boundaries that we might have bumped up against before. Strive to be steady. Steadiness says, "I will keep focused on what is important for me to do rather than spending my time and energy paying attention to anger, fear, jealousy, etc."

Steadiness comes in all forms of Fit Soul, Fit Body, and goes much deeper than keeping an athlete in a rhythm during a race to secure a win. In fact, we all seek steadiness in our everyday lives to win—to feel accomplished and in control. By feeding our bodies with the right food, we can keep blood sugar levels steady, which enables the body to be strong and allows it to devote its energies to regeneration rather than having to spend time correcting an imbalanced state. When we keep steady emotionally, we have the energy needed to cultivate our soul and fill our being with the positive attributes of life, rather than having our energies monopolized by dealing with emotional highs and lows.

Walk through life with a focus on being calm and balanced, in harmony with yourself and the world around you. The moment you feel negative thoughts or emotions robbing you of your enthusiasm, go outside to breathe in the air. Throw on some workout clothes and get some exercise. Call up a friend and make a joke about the whole situation. Shift the channel from feeling limited to becoming limitless.

Steadiness is a focus that keeps one from being pulled too deep into a negative thought or pattern. Did your motivation fall apart during a tough day at work? Remember your soul's essence, which is something good that is filled with love, energy, and the blessing of being alive. (Remember the exercise to connect with Mother Earth's love as a way to fill yourself up with this energy and feeling, page 74). Feel a sense of balance and steadiness coming from the world around you; feel yourself being connected to the world of nature and all your relatives—the four-legged ones, the winged ones, your tree ancestors, and the sky. Even in the toughest of times, the air is still giving you life. The fire, the sun and the stars, are part of your soul, giving you light. Water will quench your thirst even if you feel like life is sucking you dry. The earth is always sustaining you with her food and her love. Sit for a moment on her and nourish your being with this feeling.

These perspectives can help you feel at home on Mother Earth and enable you to keep steady no matter what is going on around you. Any given day might have gone bad, but life isn't bad! Tomorrow will be another chance to move one step closer to your goals and dreams . . . with steadiness. Close your eyes and feel your soul being part deer, part eagle as a way to remind yourself that even if life feels off-schedule, deep inside you are made of something essentially good, no matter what is going on outside. Remember your own steadiness. "I am steady in the face of challenges. I am steady in the glory of successes. My steadiness is my power. It keeps me whole and clear."

The Huichols mirror this steadiness with their emotional character and with how they approach any task. It's not that they're people without feelings—they laugh, they cry, they have emotions. But they also have a certain balance and harmony, a calmness that is interwoven with everything they do and accounts for a Huichol's stability as they move from one day to the next. Steadiness is strength for both body and soul. It means that you keep going even with bad days or weeks or months. Steadiness is a way of moving through your workouts, your life, and your challenges that says "I don't need to be able to see myself fulfilling my dream every moment for me to keep going. I will keep going even when I cannot see beyond my limits, and in this way I will surpass my limits."

How to Regain Steadiness

Here is an exercise you can use to regain your steadiness when you feel yourself being pulled away from calmness, or when you might want to throw in the towel. It can be done in a quiet place sitting down, or in the most intense, heated moment of a competition or situation in life.

- Start by remembering the nerika, the doorway or visionary circle that extends out from your heart. Imagine it just in front of you.
- Visualize yourself in the center of this sacred circle, and in that center is yourself.
- Place your focus there long enough to feel calmness rather than whatever emotion is pulling you away from your steady strength.
- Breathe in a feeling of once again being strong and feeling balanced and inspired with harmony.

Nothing outside of you has changed in that moment, but you have. This simple technique can allow your emotional strength to build and stay steady, regardless of the condition of your outer world.

Weight Lifting for the Soul

Remember that living without limits can be as simple as replacing an old pattern or way of working out with a new one that is truly effective. We have also pointed out that giving away negativity is one very potent tool for uncapping the limits and harnessing possibility as your template to live life by. This is a simple way of saying give up the worrisome thoughts that can weigh upon your soul. Lift the weight off. Give up unnecessary emotional burdens. Let your soul fly to freedom, leaving negative feelings behind. Cleanse your soul by giving away things that are holding you back from taking in the powerful medicine of good health, healing, well-being, and balance.

Of course, doing this can be challenging at times—to give up the thoughts that hold you down. But give it a try. As much as possible, try to perceive situations from a positive viewpoint. A forty-minute walk that gets shortened to twenty is still a good workout. Being calm some of the time in tough circumstances is better than never feeling peace at all. This is not to say that you have to be satisfied with the shortened workout or with a quality about yourself that you are having trouble changing. But there is something positive that can be drawn from any situation . . . always. Give yourself credit for what you did do rather than what you did not. Here are a few thoughts to bring you back to a positive outlook, one that will take you beyond limits:

Instead of "This is too hard," let the thought be "I have all it takes to make it through."

Instead of "This is a waste of time," ask yourself "What can I learn right now?"

Instead of "I don't have the time," ask yourself "How can I make my next steps a success?"

Lift the weight from your soul and let the positive aspects of life become your identity. This is the true strength of the soul.

The Four Powers

One of the themes that we keep revisiting in this book is the concept of balance, and how balance is a true asset for having a Fit Soul and a Fit Body. We emphasized this in Chapter 6, explaining the importance of having a balance of foods for health, performance, and a steady emotional state. We've given you tools to balance your physical body with aerobic exercise and strength training. Living life without limits, going to levels that were maybe only once a dream, requires having a balance of four powers that the Huichols say every single human being on this planet has and should develop to their fullest ability throughout life. The four powers are love, intuition, physical power, and the power of intelligence. If any one of these powers is missing, a person is incomplete and not capable of finding their life without limits.

We will describe each one in detail in a moment. But one of the best ways to begin to grasp what these four powers can mean to you and your life is to look at people who do not have them balanced in theirs. We need only look as far as sports figures to see what can happen when these powers are out of balance or missing in a person's life. For sure those at the top of their sport have developed physical power. But if love is missing from their lives, the thrill of victory can become a salve for an empty heart that never fills up with a love of life, which can leave an athlete groping for success well beyond his or her abilities. Without intuition guiding an athlete to success, he or she can become seduced into using drugs to bring home victory. Intelligence (in this case, living your life in the right way), if it is there, will also tell an athlete how to use his or her position for good rather than to take advantage of others. The four powers of life can transform you and give you a focused and confident outlook on life.

Let's take a look at each of these powers in more detail to see how they can help you do great things in life, and also to feel great about life.

Love

Love is the strongest of all the powers. It is said to be the foundation for developing the three others. Love is in each and every single aspect of the universe, including your body. You can have all the physical power in the world, but without love you are missing something. People who lack self-love may never have the confidence to give everything they can toward their goals. With love, a person can find the strength, steadiness, trust, and confidence to really go for their goals of body and soul. And those goals will be approached for all the right reasons. Losing weight as a way to honor one's body is very different than losing weight as a way to feel loved.

Love is much more than the sentimental concept that is glorified in movies. Love supports the body with its all-encompassing power and enables us to make the positive choices in our diet and actions that are self-supporting rather than self-defeating. Love gives you not only spiritual strength but also physical power and good thoughts about life. With love in your heart, you have the strength to do just about anything in the world. Most have experienced both sides of this. Being surrounded by a loving community that supports your efforts is extremely inspiring and can give you the motivation and energy to go to new levels of health, fitness, and well being. Coming into contact with those who despise your efforts works quite the opposite.

Embracing the power of love helps us to be better people both physically and spiritually. To love and embrace life makes us stronger on all levels. This is a reality of the soul. Having love and a Fit Soul is a foundation that is sturdy enough to help you take on the task of also having a Fit Body or physical power, which is important in any health program.

Intuition

Another spiritual power is intuition, or what many people think of as psychic power. This can evolve as having heightened awareness of yourself or your environment (what season is it, what direction are you walking or running in, which direction are you facing when you lie down at night to sleep, etc). You are using this aspect of your soul when you have feelings about things yet to happen. It's having a sense of who is calling on the phone before you look at your caller ID. It is also the part of your soul that guides you in making signifi-cant life-impacting decisions. Or if you are in a race, intuition helps you to be aware of your competitors and know what you need to do to win, if that happens to be your goal. Intuition can be thought of as your higher self, the part of you that "knows" everything already. It connects you to knowledge, wisdom, and memory—a memory of the essence of who you truly are. This is something that your being is trying to develop every moment of your life.

Cultivating your intuition, your psychic power, is a natural aspect of strength that many people in the modern world have forgotten or discounted. Everyone has psychic ability and intuitive ability. But just like how you develop your muscles, intuition is a power you have to work with to develop. How far you go with that development is personal.

When you are undecided about a bigger question in life, ask your higher self, your intuition, "What should I do?" Then listen. Listen with your heart. The answer may be what your mind is telling you to do, but it may not be. Double-check the answer with your heart, not your mind, and then act on it. We can think with our hearts as well as our minds. This is important for just about any goal or limit that you are trying to reach or go beyond. For example, the body is a very complex system and its state is affected by limitless divergent variables—the food we eat, the thoughts we tell ourselves, the environment we live in, our daily habits, exercise, etc. If you are a person who is exercising but not feeling better from it, tune in to your intuition and ask what needs to be done. The answer may have nothing to do with your exercise. It might be diet-related. It could be that you simply need more sleep, or that you're not coping well with the stress in your life. Your higher self might point out that your body feels fine, but your soul is not being nurtured. Only you will know, and you will know with intuition.

Intelligence

The third strength that relates closely to your soul is the power of intelligence. We are not talking here about the ability to outsmart someone or remember facts. The power of intelligence is living your life in the right way—being a good person, living in harmony and balance, and not abusing power. It requires learning how to treat yourself, your fellow human beings, and the earth with kindness and love. This is a strong power.

Intelligence and living your life in the right way becomes especially important to your actions when you are in a position of power. The "right way" varies from culture to culture and country to country. But certain qualities, such as honesty and integrity, are just two examples of living your life in a good way with intelligence. The list of those who have misused their status in the modern world crosses into many professions that most would consider to be immune from an abuse of this power. Using the power of intelligence to influence positive actions and bring healing is the true test of this trait.

By being intelligent you bring out the power of your soul. Living with intelligence or right action in one's life brings peace to one's soul. With it, there's nothing to feel bad or guilty about. Conversations don't have to be rearranged over and over in your mind in an attempt to feel better about their outcome. At the end of the day nothing needs to be done over or made up for. We can stand behind our actions. And this brings peace to both the soul and body.

Physical Strength

Physical strength is obviously the power that relates mostly to your body. What this means—to develop physical strength—will be different for each person. Some people have big bodies, some have little bodies, others have thin bodies, and some have not-so-thin bodies. But each one of us has a body. And regardless of body type, having a strong body helps improve muscle and joint functions, increases bone density, elevates hormone levels that can drop off with age, and most importantly creates a sense of well-being that has a profound positive effect on your outlook in life. This in turn boosts your immune system, and, in the case of people who already have chronic illnesses, can help reverse their conditions. In these ways, developing physical strength helps you to have natural resiliency of body and soul.

Having good physical strength doesn't necessarily mean having a big body with bulging muscles. Some people are built like that and are in fact very physically strong. But most of us are just average people who benefit from developing our bodies to the best of our abilities. Each person should develop his or her physical body to the best of his or her ability. What's more, developing our physical body equates with being connected to the "body" of Mother Earth. The Huichols see this as an inherent reality of body and soul. Our bodies and souls are an extension of the body and soul of Mother Earth, and this gives a person physical power.

This is the shamanic attitude toward physical strength, to do the best we can with the bodies that we have. The Huichols don't have big, burly types of bodies, but they are incredibly strong. Don José could lift a hundred pounds of firewood or corn and carry it straight up a mountain. Why? First and foremost, because he believed he could do it. Another reason is that each and every muscle in his five-foot-tall body was developed. His body was a mirror showing that size and strength are not one and the same.

Bringing the Four Powers into Your Heart

You can bring the four powers into your life with the following exercise:

- Visualize the nerika in front of your heart. Remember, this circle connects your heart to the four directions.
- Travel into this passageway, into the circle, visualizing a deer in the center.
- Visualize the deer guiding you toward the east. There in the east, look for the image of the rising sun, a bright rising sun bursting through the clouds.
- Ask the deer, your guide or your higher self, to bring one of the four powers—love, intuition, physical, or intelligence—into your circle of life from this direction. It can be any one of these four and can be different each time you do the exercise.
- When you decide which power is in this first direction, visualize it coming into your circle and the deer bringing it into your heart. Visualize love as a feeling, a feeling of being connected and embraced by all of life.

Do this with each one of three remaining directions (south, west, and north), following the deer as you travel to each one. Let the deer bring you each of the powers. In the south, visualize an eagle; in the west, water; and in the north, Mother Earth. For physical power you feel your body being connected energetically, physically, and emotionally to the body of Mother Earth. For the Huichols, this is real, not just a metaphor. When you are visualizing a connection with psychic power, think of yourself being tuned in and plugged in to the universe; you can see yourself plugged in to the core of all of creation. With intelligence, visualize or imagine a guiding force directing your every move; whether it is conscious or unconscious we can always hope to be lucky enough to make the right moves, decisions, and actions at each moment. If not, we can always try again.

By the end you will have brought each of these into your circle, into your heart, and into your life. ✤

Self-Confidence

Self-confidence means many things. For some it might be an outward bravado that looks like bragging. For others it is the ability to sit quietly, patiently, until the exact right time for making a particular move presents itself. This second example is close to the kind of self-confidence we will strive for in Fit Soul, Fit Body, one that blends steadiness, patience, and humility into a force that comes through as trusting in oneself and in life, especially life beyond our limits. Self-confidence blended with humility enables you to feel your connection to the Creator, the Great Spirit, a greater power. You are then a part of life, not separate from it.

When you are confident yet humble about your abilities (like the tortoise), you are able to experience self-proficiency without exhausting your motivation or physical strength (which is what happened to the hare). It can prevent you from continually pushing the limits just to prove that you have what it takes to go to and beyond your previous limits, or anyone else's limits, for that matter. A self-confident individual will use that ability only in the moments when it counts most. Balancing humility with self-confidence is what many people think of as positive self-esteem. It can take a lot of self-esteem to be steady yet flexible, and to be willing to let the journey of life unfold on its terms rather than trying to bend life to fit your own game plan. It takes self-confidence to allow your body to lose weight over time rather than overnight. It takes humility to keep admitting there are parts of your soul that you want to change, and to keep working to do so. It takes both to start from the beginning of a sustainable journey for body and soul, and to keep going during the rough patches until you reach the destination you seek.

Self-Doubt

Self-confidence is the positive side of the mirror that has self-doubt on the other side. Looking at the one side is empowerment for your soul. One element of what can bring self-doubt has to do with the intellectual questioning that we often go through before we even take the first step toward change. Many of us in the modern world are brought up with the "what ifs." What if I can't finish the test? What if I can't get a promotion? What if I do all this work and I'm still unhappy?

Self-doubt creates a state of mind where you spend far too much time thinking about negative things that can happen instead of focusing on the positive aspects of who you are and what you can do. You risk becoming the embodiment of your negative thoughts and derailing your quest for good health, a strong body, and a wondrous soul.

We can remedy the "what ifs" simply by taking action. Action creates joy, hope, and positive thoughts, and sustains our health and fitness goals. Scientific research has proven the positive impact taking action in the form of exercise has on your emotions. In a recent study of exercise and its effect on mood, two groups of people with histories of depression were studied. One group exercised at a moderate level of intensity (aerobic) for thirty minutes three times per week. The other group did no exercise but took medication designed to help control depression. The group that exercised had an equal reduction in the indicators of depression as the group who took the antidepressants did. More importantly, the resulting positive changes were longer lasting for the exercising group.

Honoring Life—A Recipe for Possibility

Living with self-confidence can be something of a paradox. It can require putting everything you have into an effort, but knowing it might only succeed when you can step away from that desire just enough to allow it to actually happen. True self-confidence happens when we are willing to risk it all even if it looks like we might lose everything in the process. This is possible when you are able to see your efforts as important but the results as secondary . . . the proverbial journey not the destination. And therein lies the paradox: focusing everything into our efforts without concerning ourselves with the outcome. This can be tough in the modern world with our emphasis on self, as well as results. Our world rarely rewards the journey or the effort as much as the outcome.

Here is an example of this. Picture two athletes training to win gold medals. One is self-confident and knows that the end result will be easier to swallow if she indeed brings home the medal, but that happiness will be waiting no matter what. The second athlete is also dedicating everything to this singular goal, but will be absolutely devastated if he doesn't bring home a gold medal. This mindset is lacking that deep sense of self-confidence, or even self-respect. But as we all know, life works out quite well for lots of people who don't win gold medals! Which one do you think has a better chance of actually winning it?

Clearly the first one. Knowing life will work out (self-confidence) often frees us up to actually accomplish the big dreams beyond our normal limits. And this can begin by honoring all of life, which is another way of having trust in it.

The directive to "honor all life" can release you from the restraints of too much personal introspection or self-importance. Honoring life can allow you to lift yourself up and look outward into the limitless possibility reflected in the natural world. It's possible to achieve success in all aspects of our life—from physical health to emotional and spiritual well-being. We can also feel assured that we are not the first ones embarking on this path to wholeness. Others have come before us and have succeeded, and others will succeed in the future. Therefore, we can say that we are a reflection of the miraculous success of the universe in sustaining life on this planet and beyond. We as humans should remember this in our striving for health, balance, and overall wellness. "We are a mirror of the ancient ones, our ancient ancestors," say the Huichols over and over again.

This is one goal or objective of shamanism. You are a part of all that exists. We all breathe the air no matter where we are. We all walk upon the earth. Even if there is cement at our feet, there is still Mother Earth below. There is still Father Sky above us. As a human being, you are in the middle. You are a medium between earth and sky, a bridge between the worlds. This is a bigger version of how we feel when we are part of a workout group or a spiritual group, to be part of a big family rather than alone or on the outside of something great that is going on.

Honoring life starts with simple statements about how you want to live your life. "I want to live. I want be a part of life. I want to be a part of the rivers that flow into the ocean. I want to be a part of the beautiful Grandmother Ocean that washes over the sand before me and inside of my being. I want to be a part of the exquisite sunrise and the sunset, to be aware of the sky above and the earth below. I honor the spirit of creation. I honor the spirits of nature. This is who I am as a human being."

Here is a powerful instruction or meditation that you can use to help make this connection to wholeness; you learned a version of this earlier in the book:

Sit in a quiet place and feel, visualize, or imagine a cord from the bottom of your spine going down into Mother Earth. Feel as if your body is an extension of the body of Mother Earth. As you breathe slowly, feel as if you are breathing in all the beauty that sits on Mother Earth: the beautiful mountains, lakes, waterfalls, anything that you feel is beautiful and powerful.

You may visualize yourself flying with a bird or flowing down a river. Either way, you are moving through life finding wholeness and a connection to your environment. This is an exercise any person can do anytime to increase strength or your ability to feel whole.

Life without Limits Begins with You

Living beyond limits, life without borders can be as easy as trying a new activity, being more steady in your efforts, gaining self-confidence by feeling confident in life itself. It can be as challenging as finding a new positive spin on an old situation that normally brings you negative thoughts. It can be as daunting as saying, yes I might fail, but I will try anyway. Life without limits begins with you, is supported through community, and can take all four powers (love, physical, intuitive, intelligence) to accomplish. But remember, a seed can become a redwood, the sun was once a young girl, and you in a few tomorrows can become that vision that exists beyond today's limits. ☙

Chapter Eight
A Fit Vision for Life

No puzzle is too great for the Great Spirit to solve . . .

We have shared with you many tools for bringing Fit Soul, Fit Body alive. In my own life, there was perhaps no greater example of how much impact bringing these two worlds together can have than the yearlong journey to the final Ironman of my career in 1995. As I mentioned in the very first chapter, my time as Brant's student changed me from being an athlete with a spiritual approach to life to being a spiritual person who also did athletics, and who used having a Fit Soul as the foundation that enabled me to do everything from getting out the door each day for training all the way up to winning races. I saw others in my sport struggling for life's answers by fine-tuning their intervals on the track or maybe adding a new race into their schedule, hoping it would bring them success, happiness, and a sense of fulfillment.

I was lucky enough from my very first retreat with Brant in Mexico to see that those results in races could be part of feeling satisfied in life, but certainly were not the underlying avenue that would take me to a place of peace in a sustainable way. This was something that became absolutely clear after my third win in Kona. The incredible feeling of accomplishment and fulfillment lasted almost a year after my first victory in 1989, the second one lasted about three months, and then the third a few weeks. The light bulb went on when I asked myself how many Ironman victories I would need to win to feel good about life each and every day. A hundred? A thousand? This was a major turning point between my athletic and spiritual focus, from hoping a fit body would sustain my soul to making sure my soul was intact . . . then using that strength to tend to my body.

I had experienced an incredible feeling of joy and contentment the first time I went with Brant to a retreat. Each time after that brought those same feelings deeper into my heart and lasted longer. The wisdom of his words helped wash away patterns and thoughts that got in my way of connecting with real peace. His ceremonies balanced my being and seemed to be changing me even on a cellular level. Each time I did the exercises (like the ones you have in this book) something good happened. It might be making a new connection to the world of nature that gave me strength, or a nugget of wisdom, or just a sense of well-being that put all of life's problems in perspective and brought me happiness. Simple yet powerful.

I was lucky . . . extremely lucky. I could have struggled through a never-ending number of attempts to win the Ironman, but certainly I would have never been able to do so without Brant and the Huichol tradition. And even if I had somehow won without his immense help, support, and power, I still would not have been able to find real peace, the kind that is not fleeting. I found a teacher with compassion, wisdom, power, and a healing energy that brought all things in the world and in my life into alignment. I'd seen others have great successes in various sports, only to later be disillusioned when those moments didn't sustain them for life. In desperation, they would try going back to drink from the waters of victory long after the well had dried up.

My time was coming. No athlete can be at the top of his or her sport forever. 1995 was going to be farewell, my final Ironman . . . win, lose, or draw. Certainly a win was the goal. Yet by 1995 there were several huge roadblocks that could have taken my dream and turn it into a nightmare. First, I would be thirty-seven years old by race day, placing me solidly outside the golden years for winning at that event. No one had ever been victorious who was anywhere close to being that old. On any given day I was going to have to trim my workouts back 25 to 50 percent from previous levels, simply because I was too old to absorb the high volume of training I had done in the past.

Secondly, no matter how much balance one strives for in elite athletics, there is always a price to be paid. For me it was that my body was getting tired and my reserves were running low, which is a bad combination for someone trying to pull off the impossible. In addition, I was going to be racing athletes ten to fifteen years younger, who could put in the real Ironman training necessary, at least on the physical level. I would be trying to beat guys that I had not finished ahead of in almost two years. On paper there was absolutely zero percent chance that I could win, even with my experience.

But Brant had said to me so many times in the years leading up to this race: "No puzzle is too great for the Great Spirit to solve." I knew I could count on Brant to help me develop a Fit Soul and to do everything in a shaman's power to bring my depleted body back into balance. Without a Fit Soul, my thirty-seven-year-old body would unquestionably come up short. Without his help I would have certainly succumbed to self-doubt even before I took my first step training. Without Brant my fear of the age factor would have eroded my self-confidence and led me to do too much training out of desperation. Without his ceremonies to get the Ancient Ones, the elemental powers, involved in helping me, I would have arrived in Kona just like every other champion who was grasping for one too many victories. But fortunately, another destiny would play out.

Mind and Soul Over Matter

I moderated my training as a thirty-seven-year-old, letting the young guys win the daily workouts. I skipped a lot of sessions simply because I was still feeling tired and knew I would need every ounce of reserve energy I could store up for race day. I saw Brant a few extra times that year, trying to focus as much of my energy as possible to gain a truly Fit Soul. In August, right at the time when my training partners were in the thick of their Ironman training, I went to Brant's annual summer retreat. This particular year it was eight days in the wilds of Alaska. It would signal the first turning point for the better that happened to me all year.

When Brant first saw me, he immediately asked, "Are you going to win the Ironman this year?" My response was, "Are you going to help me?" He gave me the shaman's once-over to assess my situation and said, "You need some extra help this year!" That was the last we spoke about Ironman for those eight wonderful days immersed in the natural beauty and power of Alaska. No alarm clock needed— just wait for the eagles to sing and the whales to sound the start of a new day!

Brant used that time to have me do all of the same exercises I had done over and over before. He spoke words that would later bring me out of desperate moments in the race, which was coming up in two months' time. He took me to places of power to leave offerings and prayers, and to call out with positive affirmations as a way to ask for what was important in my life. While my training partners were home doing long workouts, hoping to gain strength, Brant did special healing ceremonies to bring my body back into balance and to charge it up with energy. The rest of my competitors were searching their logbooks for the answers to victory. I was finding those answers immersed in the natural power of Alaska, focusing on having a Fit Soul.

One of Brant's final instructions for me was to make sure to stop in Central California where he lived on my way to the Ironman, so that he could do one more ceremony to get me ready. I had learned just a few weeks earlier from a blood test that my internal chemistry looked more like that of a sixty-year-old than someone in their mid-thirties. Not a good state for someone trying to win an Ironman! Brant tuned right in to this. In his wisdom, he knew that even a week in Alaska wasn't going to be enough to bring me completely back, and that more would be needed. I had never made this extra effort before, but even though I now felt ready, I also knew that his intuition was to be trusted completely.

My training did start to come around when I got back from the retreat. I found myself easily leading workouts that I had been struggling to keep up with before going to Alaska. My confidence was soaring for the race closing in. I also knew that it could be a test like no other, and that my final preparation would come in the last blessing from Brant on my way to the race.

A ceremonial fire was going outside his home when I arrived, that beautiful light that people all around the earth have gathered around for millennia. A few quick moments of joking to ease the tension that was building about what was ahead of me in Hawaii, and then on to the work of a shaman. Brant chanted his sacred songs that took my heart to a place of hope, trust, and joy. He worked in a way that very few on this planet could to arrange help for me from the elemental powers that the Huichols have honored since time began. He gave my body strength and power in a natural way, using his songs. The final moment was confirmed with a handshake, a hug, and a look in his eyes that said I was ready.

Thirty-seven is not especially old by most measures. But in the world of elite athletics, I was ancient, I was a fossil, and all the young guys were salivating at this final and most likely good chance to chew me up and spit me out all over that lava. In previous years, I was Mark Allen the returning champion . . . a fact that I could exploit to my advantage in the race. But now I was Mark Allen the aging vet coming back for what most of my competitors hoped would be one too many. There was not one look of being intimidated from any of them. It was like limping into a pack of hungry wolves. No hope for escape.

The Race of a Lifetime

At 7:00 A.M. the starting cannon sounded the beginning of a day that no one knows what it will take to finish. Fifty minutes later, I exited the swim and had my first real gauge of how the day was unfolding. On the way to my bike I was told that most of my top competitors were still in the water . . . certainly a great sign. I breathed a small sigh of relief. Even a few seconds' advantage on the bike can be enough to slip out of sight and out of mind. An unseen leader is always tougher to beat than a competitor at your side who you can size up moment by moment.

The bike portion of the race started better than I could have imagined. At only fifteen miles into it, and with ninety-seven to go, I took the lead. My heart rate was well within my limits, I felt fantastic, and I was at the front of the race earlier than I had been at any of my other Ironman victories. At that exact moment I made my first mistake. I started thinking how easy this final win was going to be, and felt that surge of overconfidence that takes one away from a steady point of being alert and clear. As you have read, Brant emphasizes how the Huichols strive to be steady: never too up and certainly never too down. They focus on steadiness to bring them strength so that they don't become like a yo-yo going from highs to lows and back again. Well, I let myself forget this powerful teaching and found myself already assembling the acceptance speech I would give the following night at the awards ceremony.

Ironman has a million ways to bring you back down to reality. This year it was going to come in the form of a twenty-four-year-old German soldier named Thomas Hellriegel, who passed me looking like he was on a motorcycle. He never looked back. By the end of the bike segment, he had amassed a lead of over thirteen minutes. With a marathon staring me in the face, I knew that to have any chance of winning I would need to take thirty seconds a mile out of him, every single mile of the run. And this certainly sounded completely impossible. No one had ever come back from that far down to win.

"No puzzle is too great for the Great Spirit to solve." Brant's words brought hope to my soul, giving me the confidence to at least start the marathon. There were a thousand moments in the opening miles of the run when I wanted to just call it quits. "I've won five titles. That's enough, isn't it? Who needs this kind of pain and humiliation? I certainly don't!"

A few miles in and no time gained. The course crossed directly in front of my hotel. It was now or never. Quit or keep going. Quitting would be easy. Keeping going sounded impossible. "It's never over until it's over," another philosophy the Huichols live by that Brant had said over and over again, came back to me. If I quit, there was certainly no hope of winning. If I took the easy way out, there was no hope that everything Brant had done to help me be ready could work. If I could keep myself going, there might be a chance.

"The Ancient Ones always test our intentions," Brant would tell us as we sat in a circle around the fire. I was beginning to get a firsthand experience of what this meant. I certainly wanted to win, but had an image of it happening in a nice, easy way. The reality of this goal as it unfolded was total chaos. It didn't match any nice and tidy pre-race plan I had for the day. But there was still hope. Brant had arranged everything for my body and soul to be ready. It was now my job to live what I had asked for by keeping going, and to honor my teacher, his work, and the Huichol tradition.

A mile later I passed my first competitor and moved into third place. Nearly thirteen miles after that I worked my way into second. Now there was only one person standing between me and victory. The gap was narrowing at nearly thirty seconds per mile. But it was far from enough to guarantee the dream I was after.

Five miles later with eight to go, a four-minute gap stood between the victory and me. What transpired in the next fifty minutes would label my career forever. If I pulled it off, I would be remembered as one of the greatest in the sport. If I fell short, I wouldn't be remembered as the five-time Ironman champ, but rather as the old guy who came back for one too many. Pressure? Just a little.

"Everything is alive . . . the trees, the stones, the earth. Call out when you need help." Brant emphasized this over and over in every seminar and retreat I ever participated in with him. The Big Island is certainly alive. Standing over 30,000 feet tall from its base at the ocean floor to its highest point atop Mauna Kea, its power is undeniable. I called out. "Help me! I'm going to give it everything I have. But I need your help."

The next mile I made up about forty seconds on Hellriegel, the one after that over fifty seconds, and the one after that a minute and fifteen seconds. At mile twenty-three of the marathon, I finally caught the leader, who had once been thirteen minutes ahead and was still thirteen years younger. Three miles after that I closed out my Ironman career with a sixth World Championship title in a race that would go down as the greatest comeback in Ironman history.

My first six years racing the Ironman in Hawaii were spent struggling, never finding answers to a question that I didn't even know I needed to ask: how to have a Fit Soul. The second six came about by having the good luck to meet Brant and study with him. His blessings, healings, and teachings brought life to my spirit and made me stronger on all the levels that had plagued me with weakness. His guidance as a teacher and his friendship helped me develop a Fit Soul, which became the essence that brought my dreams into form with six Ironman titles and a life that is filled with simple tools that create profound change.

I continue to study with him to this day, using the same practices that you have in this book as a way to continue my journey of Fit Soul, Fit Body for life. I take time away from my everyday life to plug back in to the world of nature at his retreats around the world in wondrous places like the Island of Crete in Greece, the Italian Alps, Alaska, Mount Shasta, and Japan. I also make it a daily ritual to do many of the exercises you have right here in this book. Each small step adds up to big transformations over time. Fit Soul, Fit Body for life is a goal worthy of us all.

Just One Approach to Many Lofty Goals

As you have seen, Fit Soul, Fit Body can be used to help you improve yourself physically, emotionally, and spiritually. It can help you to achieve whatever goals you set for yourself, be they goals related to your professional path, relationships, health, or athletic pursuits. The exercises for your body and the practices for your soul are for everyone, whether you live in a Huichol village in Mexico or in an apartment building in a big city. As we have emphasized, these exercises and perspectives work over time. There is no quick fix. Sudden fitness or weight loss will only be short-lived. The big changes in our personality and soul take more commitment than a weekend's worth of work. Transformations that are enduring are rarely noticeable moment to moment. It's usually not until you look back after a few months or a few years of steady work that you see the dramatic changes.

This is why we refer to Fit Soul, Fit Body as a "journey for life." Use this concept—evolve over time—to make your life a wondrous journey. One run won't enable you to lose all the extra weight. Consistent running over time likely will. Then, once you get there, stick with your program so the change is permanent. Likewise, learning Fit Soul exercises won't prevent you from facing new challenges and having disappointments in the future. But consistently practicing those exercises will allow you to move more freely through difficult times. Commit to a day-to-day shift away from old patterns that do not serve you. Adopt the ones that do and use them in your approach to dealing with the world for the rest of your life.

To ensure that Fit Soul, Fit Body is a journey for your entire life, continue to adopt and use the exercises in this book. Once you have achieved the immediate goals you establish, adjust and rethink your next steps for the long term. In the rest of this chapter, we will discuss your evolving goals, and the tools you will need to achieve them while giving your soul purpose, maintaining balance, and experiencing *you*. Many of the ideas presented here reinforce and expand upon concepts previously covered.

The Evolving Fit Body Goal

In Chapter 4 we showed how you could use a particular goal to get started on your program and also use that goal to help sustain motivation over time. But what happens when you get to the end point? When you get what you want, what next?

A lot of people just stop. The goal has been accomplished, but doing it all over again just doesn't have the pizzazz it had the first time around. This question becomes most important to have an answer to when the most immediate goal is one that may possibly never be achievable again. Let's face facts. Some goals, especially physical ones like winning Ironmans, have a shelf life. We will not be able to get faster, go longer, or become stronger forever, especially when we reach the twilight years of our life. If you are searching for the next step in your Fit Body journey, here are a few evolving goals that may help keep you going:

- **Keep consistent**. We keep mentioning this because it's so important. All good things come from consistency. And all goals, both for body and soul, come about with consistency in working toward them. If the distances you have been keeping up have become a stress producer instead of a stress reliever, rather than giving up, start cutting them back by 10 to 15 percent a week until you find a level that gives you that good feeling again—in your body as well as your soul.

- **Mix it up**. Try a new sport, or an old one that you haven't done for a while. In either case, you will almost certainly experience that feeling of getting better and gaining proficiency for a long period. Just keep in mind that if it's a sport you did twenty years ago, your expectations of what you can do now may need to be adjusted to match your current age. You can also "mix it up" by engaging in new activities and groups, or by taking a new class to expand your knowledge about a subject that interests you. There are a million ways to mix it up, and find fresh sources of motivation and inspiration to fuel your Fit Soul, Fit Body visions.

- **Share your experience**. Teach someone else how to do what you have become good at. There's no greater thrill than seeing someone experience the joy you felt in the opening years of your own learning curve.

- **Look around you**. Set goals based on your peer group. Particularly if you feel your body getting older, instead of focusing on achieving a personal best in a particular event, try focusing on moving up in the ranks among your peers instead. They are getting older (and probably slower) too, so it might be good to forget about the actual race time and go for a better placing.

- **Keep making deposits**. View your health as a bank account that should always be tended to. Every day you are sedentary, a small withdrawal is made on it. Every day you exercise, you become a littler richer.

Giving Your Soul Purpose

We have just as much—if not more—responsibility to take care of our soul as we do our body. This is where that thing called "you" begins. And the "you" that you are today wants to continue to grow every day of your life, whether you feel this desire in the moment or not. Here is a job for your soul to do in each season so that you can continually be a part of your world and its changing moods, and to

An Aging Body Can Still Be a Fit Body

There is no age that is too old to start a fitness program, or even to become a shaman, and certainly never a time to trade in the athletic shoes and a sharp mind for a soft chair and a dull life. A prime example of this was my adopted grandfather, Don José, who lived to be 110 years old, and up until his final two years could carry heavy loads up and down the hillsides in his homeland. Your immediate fitness goals will change as you evolve and age. But by revisiting your goals, sticking to a workout program, and paying attention to your soul, you can ensure you have a fit body and soul for life. ✿

help your soul feel in sync and alert throughout each year of your life.

Winter is a time of regeneration. Just as the earth is resting and regenerating, think of this as a time to regenerate your body and soul. Take the light of the sun and the fire and draw it inside your heart as a way to reflect on your life. Plants draw on this light, pulling their life force inside during the fall, and then using the winter to regenerate their essence. You can visualize that process of regeneration going on inside of your own body at this time of year.

When spring comes, reflect on the waking up of the earth with the same feeling inside of you. This can be a period where you "come alive," waking up renewed and emerging from the dream-state of winter.

As summer returns, shift again, feeling yourself filled with the light of the season of light. Celebrate the summer. Celebrate the light.

With fall, it's a time to reflect, to once again start going inside, and to harvest all of the light of the summer. It's a season to harvest your enthusiasm, and to harvest all that you've experienced and learned in the other seasons. Hold these things inside so that, as the seasons and years go by, you are still caught up in the beauty of your program and your goals of Fit Soul, Fit Body. This is a way to rediscover your soul each year of your journey.

Humans respond well to variations throughout the year. It's absolutely essential to keep this in mind in your workout routine, and in everyday life as well. For example, vary your physical activity volume (your weekly total hours of exercise), the length of your longest days, the activities you choose, and the level of intensity and adherence you have to daily working out. Just as a person would crave a little rain if every day were sunny, our bodies crave something different if we fed it the same exercise every day of the year. Having variation brings about positive responses and changes.

Life as a Circle

We often think of a journey as a straight line that leads from one point to another, and in a sense it is. We start a task and hopefully at some point we complete it. That is a straight line. But it is also a circle. A circle connects the past, the present, and the future. The circle is a sacred symbol of unity, connecting us to all of life. Life doesn't just stop. There is always a point that lies beyond the step you are taking in this moment. There is always a season that lies beyond the current one. With the completion of one year, another one begins. There will always be a sunrise that lies beyond the current sunset.

Allow the completion of one step lead you to the beginning of the next one. An example of this is someone who might choose a marathon as the big goal to draw them into the action of training. They may devote a year to complete this goal, and when it finally comes, the feeling can be something that leaves an incredibly positive impression on that person's soul. This brings them back to the beginning of being ready to continue on with the next step on their journey. Let your life be a reflection of this in all that you do, evolving your goals and purpose as you go, always searching for the next step and then taking it.

Life is seen this way in Huichol cosmology. By going on pilgrimages, by walking on Mother Earth to sacred places of power, the Huichols see themselves as reliving creation. And so they are beginning anew throughout their entire lives. This is living Fit Soul, Fit Body. This concept, life as a circle, is what can give us strength to continue on during the trials that come up. We have all had to go through times when our personal tests seem endless. But there will always be a point when it comes full circle and you finally make it through the test. Ride it out! Let your soul shine in the midst of calamity or challenge. Reflect calm in the middle of doubt. Make the changes in your daily routines and approach to life that brings satisfaction and joy to your soul. Trust in yourself, in uncertainty, in the universe.

An ultimate goal for body and soul from a Huichol perspective is to live our life in harmony and balance with ourselves, our community, and all of life on Mother Earth. We could furthermore say this is to become a reflection of our ancient ancestors, learning from the lives of others who have gone before us, whether they are in our own personal family or not, and also learning from the spirit of nature. A simple understanding of this could be not building your house in a place where a river often overflows. We have learned how to reflect on the ways of indigenous peoples, to eat good foods that do not pollute our bodies. A positive image for a Huichol is to imagine food, air, and water empowering the body every day. Once again we are feeding our soul as we are connecting our bodies to life surrounding us, helping us feel a part of the circle of life.

Maintaining Balance

Each step you take on your journey of Fit Soul, Fit Body takes you closer to being balanced, being more fit, having better overall health and a better attitude toward life, being able to feel peaceful and at home in just about any situation. We often forget to notice and give thanks when our body and soul are in balance because this natural state lacks the signs of being out of balance: having an illness, being injured, having anger, fear, or jealousy, being burned out, feeling unmotivated or stressed. Unfortunately, these negative situations are often the ones that make us sit up and take notice.

This can then be part of your journey for life—notice the subtlety that exists in balance. Notice that negative thoughts are not present when you have a positive outlook, or at least when negativity is kept at bay. Notice that the sun rose yesterday and that it set last night. Notice that you have been consistent in your workouts. Pay attention to how good you feel when you are active. Don't wait until you can't move your body to realize how important it is for your life. Acknowledge yourself for your efforts when you feel balanced. Use the tools to maintain balance before it becomes a disaster that tells you it's time to do something about your life.

Balanced or Not?

Here is a short checklist of both being in balance and being out. If the out of balance describes your current state, it might be time to reevaluate and make some significant changes so that Fit Soul, Fit Body has a chance of surviving and being a part of your life. Remember to go back to the quiz in Chapter 1 whenever you like; it's a great way to check in with yourself and see how you're doing, especially if you sense that you've fallen off track.

Balanced:

- You wake up excited and happy for the day.
- You have time for others.
- You have witnessed some aspect of nature in the last twenty-four hours.
- There is little nagging worry on your mind.
- You feel motivated more often than not.
- There is measurable improvement in fitness and health markers.
- You are injury-free and live an active life.

Out of Balance:

- You would rather pull the sheets over your head than march out the door to tackle the day.
  Solution: If this is your overwhelming feeling, it might be a good idea to take a break and have some down time. Rest is just as important as action.
- There is always a burning feeling of stress or anxiety that just won't go away.
  Solution: Do the Fit Soul Exercise for Trust on page 103.
- You can hardly stand it when people want to talk with you or need your help because you are barely able to take care of your own life.

Solution: Take some moments to disconnect from whatever gives you the stress and do something positive for yourself. Take a short walk, watch the sunset, or breathe in the aroma and exquisite colors of a flower—anything to reset the positive meter. In other words, find and nurture your higher self.

- Nature? Who has the time for nature?!

  Solution: Remember how we are all set up, which is to find good health, solace, and joy in the events that are taking place each and every day, which also took place before the modern world.

- You have ongoing injuries and/or frequent illnesses that recur or just don't seem to go away.

  Solution: Cut back both the volume and intensity of your training. Do a life stress reality check and do what you can to reduce the overall load. Dedicate yourself to doing some of the key Fit Soul exercises that counter any stresses in life and fill you up personally with a feeling of energy.

- You feel too overwhelmed or lack the motivation to exercise.

  Solution: Look at the big picture. Do what you can to clear your plate a little bit so there is time. Plug in to your community of support for help and motivation.

- You cannot make any gains in fitness.

  Solution: Vary the routine. If what you have been doing isn't working, change can stimulate your body to go forward once again. Also do a reality check to make sure that your efforts are in line with your goals.

Experiencing You

Often trying to become something that we are not is what gets us out of balance in the first place. Not everyone is built to win races or become a healer. Honoring what is right for each of us is what keeps us on track and has value in the world.

One's true nature can be tough to get a feel for in the modern world. With job responsibilities, advertisements for bodies that only 1 percent of the population will ever be able to achieve, and an overall pace that offers little time to reflect on what is important, it can all add up to striving for goals that are not necessarily reflections of our true calling in either our physical fitness or in the pursuits we undertake to bring joy to our souls. This can take us out of balance as we follow goals and dreams that are not coming from inside ourselves.

The Huichols offer very effective tools that can help you tune back in to what is important, realistic, and right for you. It is called living through the heart. Living through the heart takes the modern-world influences out of the equation when we need the answer to two very important questions: Who am I, and what is right for me to do in my journey of body and soul?

Living through the heart requires experiencing rather than analyzing our world. Your heart is the part of your awareness that gives you thoughts and answers to life when you are not focused on them. Living through your heart is that gentle force nudging you toward a purpose, which your logical thoughts may not understand at this moment. Whether we are in need of reevaluating our health goals or our purpose in life, this is a way of really knowing what is important, because it takes the mind out of coming up with the answer and enables a person to feel his or her true nature. The mind is the part of you that analyzes and interprets everything as good or bad, right or wrong, and puts labels on life that can come from external influences and standards. By approaching workouts, life, and your connection to community and the world of nature through your heart, you will have a better sense of knowing what is right, sustainable, and in tune with the real you.

Experiencing the World with Your Heart Exercise

Here are images that you can use this very moment to begin experiencing your world with your heart.

With every breath you take, try to feel your heart opening. Feel yourself being connected to and becoming aware of your inner and outer environments at the same time.

Feel how your heart is connecting to and perceiving your outer environment. You have to use your own inner guidance in doing this and to move your focus away from anything that might be distracting you. Are you aware of the world in front of you, or are you lost in your thoughts? Can you see something with natural beauty, or is your mind blinding you with chatter?

Make the shift. Ask your higher self—or as the Huichols say, ask the deer spirit of your heart—to help you do this. Feel how your heart is not only an organ inside of your body, but also a means of connecting you to the world. How do you do this? By trusting your feelings. Trust your own awareness and your relationship to your environment and the world around you. By connecting to your outer world with your heart, what you see shifts from being an exercise in taking inventory of the world to feeling a positive emotion that comes from being touched by its beauty, wonder, and magnificence.

Visualize your personal well-being coming into fruition by opening your heart, by opening your essence, by opening the very core of your being. You are then creating your reality. And when you have this reality there is no place for the other. 🐾

Opening your heart to good thoughts and visualizing light coming into your own heart is a way to wash away stress and other negative emotions. Opening your heart and soul to positive feelings gives a place for your true essence and calling in life to be experienced.

A Vision for Life

A Fit Soul and Fit Body are two diverse but intrinsically connected aspects of your being that this book can help you nourish. We hope that you have been inspired and encouraged to bring these worlds together. Let them empower you. Become a whole, happy, joyous being. Build the strength and health of your body. There is a fit life that is right for you. Let food be medicine for your body. Let life be medicine for your soul.

Come into the light. Become a part of the four seasons. Feel the love of the earth. Be a part of the conscious breathing organism that

Don José's Metaphor for an Open Heart

Don José taught me about opening the heart with a simple metaphor. When I asked him about light and darkness, and about different realities, he told me, "Close the door, grandson." I closed the door to his small home. The house was in complete darkness. (There are no windows in a traditional Huichol house; the only opening is the door.) Then he pushed open the door and said, "Look, you can see now, can't you?" because of course the house was flooded with light. Don José said, "This is the way your heart is. Open the door, open the heart and let the light in, and then there is no place for darkness."

is the earth. Let your heart be overwhelmed with her love. Let yourself be washed with the beauty of nature. Live what truly has meaning for you in your heart. The colors of a beautiful sunset can bring a sense of well-being to your soul. Witnessing a thousand sunsets can change your perspective and your soul forever.

Each day on this journey will be different, just as every single sunrise is different. There is never a point where you arrive and that is it. It's a path inviting you to walk on it every day of your life. Each day is a chance to rededicate yourself to living life with joy, happiness, and power as a whole human being. Transform what holds you back. Rediscover your enthusiasm by taking in the light and living through your heart. Don José emphasized that we are just who we are at any given moment in our lives. "If you fall down," he said, "stand up and keep going." This can be your inspiration . . . the words of a great shaman who lived a wondrous life for 110 years.

Never underestimate your joy, your power, or your capabilities. Keep going even when you feel you are not able to go on. Trust in the Great Mystery that is working behind all the events in life. Bring laughter into your community. Draw hope into your heart and live an existence that nurtures your soul and your body. The living principles of Fit Soul, Fit Body are for you and everyone to use.

Huichol Prayer Offering

"Great Spirit, Grandfather Fire, Mother Earth, Father Sky, I offer you my life. Give me peace. Open my heart. Show me what it means to love my life and to love all of life. Help me reflect you with each step I take on this beautiful altar of Mother Earth." ✾

About the Authors

Brant Secunda is a shaman-healer in the Huichol tradition of Mexico. He completed a 12-year apprenticeship with the legendary Huichol shaman Don José Matsuwa. Brant is the director of the Dance of the Deer Foundation Center for Shamanic Studies and teaches seminars and retreats worldwide.

For more information on Brant, go to shamanism.com.

Mark Allen is a six-time Ironman Triathlon World Champion. He was named Triathlete of the Year six times by *Triathlete* magazine and called "The World's Fittest Man" by *Outside* magazine. Mark's final victory in 1995 at age 37 makes him the oldest men's champion in the history of the race. Mark attributes his Ironman dominance to Brant's teachings, ceremonies and healings. Mark continues to study with Brant to this day.

For more information on Mark, visit markallenonline.com.

Fit Soul, Fit Body began as a seminar organized by Brant and Mark more than a decade ago. They have presented it worldwide, and it served as the inspiration for this book.

❀

*For more information, please visit
fitsoul-fitbody.com.*